Massage
for
Healthier
Children

Massage
for
Healthier
Children

Marybetts Sinclair
Illustrations by Richard Robertson

Wingbow Press
Oakland, California

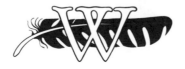

Manufactured in the United States of America.

Wingbow Press books are published and distributed by Bookpeople, 7900 Edgewater Drive, Oakland, California 94621.

Library of Congress Cataloging-in-Publication Data:
    Sinclair, Marybetts.
    Massage for healthier children / Marybetts Sinclair; illustrations by Richard Robertson.
        p. cm.
    Includes bibliographical references and index.
    ISBN 0-914728-76-8   92-11050
    1. Massage for children. I. Title.
    RJ53.M35S56 1992
    615.8'22—dc20

Design by Brenn Lea Pearson.
Cover photo by Laurence Brun—Agence Rapho.
Author photo by Ball Studio, Corvallis, Oregon.
Photo on page 66 courtesy of Dr. Robert Toporek.

This book is designed for use by lay persons, not as a substitute for bodywork training. It is not intended for the purpose of diagnosing, or as a substitute for medical treatment, and does not take responsibility for readers' use of the information herein.

First printing October 1992

Grateful acknowledgement is made to the following for permission to reprint previously published material:
Cartoon by Jim Borgman, copyright © 1991 by King Features. Reprinted with special permission of King Features Syndicate, Inc.
"Touching and Being Touched" by Robert Coles, appearing in *The Dial*, December 1980. Reprinted by permission of Professor Coles.
"Relaxation Therapy in Asthma: A Critical Review," by Erskine-Miliss and Schonell, appearing in *Psychosomatic Medicine*, pp. 365-70, August 1981. Copyright © 1981 by American Psychosomatic Society.
Cartoon by Nicole Hollander, copyright © 1985 Nicole Hollander. Reprinted with permission.
Stress in Childhood, edited by James H. Humphrey. Reprinted by permission of AMS Press, Inc. Copyright © 1984 by AMS Press, Inc.
Cholesterol and Children by Robert E. Kowalski. Copyright © 1988 by Robert E. Kowalski. Reprinted with the permission of HarperCollins.
Spinning Inward by Maureen Murdock. © 1987 by Maureen Murdock. Reprinted by arrangement with Shambhala Publications, Inc., 300 Massachusetts Ave., Boston, MA 02115.
Take Care of Your Child by Pantell, Fries and Vickery, © 1990 by Addison-Wesley Publishing Company, Inc. Reprinted by permission of the publisher.
High Tech Touch by Jeanne St. John. Copyright © 1987 by Academic Therapy Publications. Reprinted by permission of Academic Therapy Publications, 20 Commercial Blvd., Novato, CA 94949.
"Massage Therapy—Who Kneads It?" by T.C. Hunter, appearing in *Arthritis Today*, March-April 1991. Copyright © 1991 by T.C. Hunter.
"The significance of life events as contributing factors in the diseases of children," appearing in *Journal of Pediatrics*. Copyright © 1973 by *Journal of Pediatrics*.
"Children Under Stress" by Beth Brothy with Maureen Walsh, appearing in *U.S. News and World Report*. Copyright © 1986 by *U.S. News and World Report*.

To David Werner and Meir Schneider,
in appreciation of their compassion, insight,
and dedication to the welfare of others.

Contents

Foreword

Recent research confirms what many massage therapists have reported: that massage helps the growth and development of children. Studies in our lab, for example, suggest that massage helps growth in young infants and reduces stress in older children. In one study, preterm infants in incubators gained 47 percent more weight when they were massaged. They also became more responsive to social stimulation and showed better motor development. Later in the first year of life they were still showing a growth and cognitive motor development advantage. In another study we massaged children who were hospitalized for psychiatric problems. Those children, who were normally deprived of touch, showed several improvements. Their sleep improved, they were less anxious and agitated, and their cortisol and norepinephrine levels—biochemical indicators of stress—decreased.

Marybetts Sinclair's *Massage for Healthier Children* suggests that all children—both normal and those with special needs—can benefit from massage. It beautifully expresses the value of massage for closeness, comfort and relaxation; it outlines the importance of "what your hands say;" and it describes a full body massage technique. Several of the massage strokes are also nicely illustrated. These "how to" chapters are followed by chapters on healing common discomforts of the normal child and massaging the special needs child. These are the unique features of this book.

A bibliography and a list of resources complete this comprehensive, well designed and clearly written book. I am sure this volume will be very useful for massage therapists, and parents would love having these lessons on how to massage their children.

Tiffany Field, Ph.D.
Professor of Pediatrics and Psychology
University of Miami School of Medicine

Preface

I began my career as a massage therapist by working with normal healthy
adults, and found that massage was a
wonderful way for them to relax and feel
nurtured. Later I massaged many people
with more specific needs, and was delighted
to discover the great benefits massage had
for them as well. Among those who deeply
appreciated massage were pregnant women,
mothers in labor, rape victims, invalids, and
those suffering from chronic pain, physical
handicaps, or terminal illnesses. I was able
to help people spontaneously in situations
such as a tension headache at a party,
menstrual cramps at a dance class, or low
back pain on a hiking trip. I provided
massage for all ages, from babies a few
minutes old to people in their nineties. I
massaged the very wealthy and the desper-
ately poor. As my experience increased, my
opinion of massage became higher and
higher. The positive response to a caring,
sensitive massage seemed universal.

Recipients of massage feel looser and
more flexible; they can breathe and move
more freely, and they are more emotionally
and mentally relaxed. People love massage
for all these reasons, and because it gives
them an interval of peace and quiet which
is rare in our culture. Massage can also
teach the ability to consciously relax—a
skill most of us never learned as children.

Massage cannot cure the chronic pain of
conditions like polio, cancer or arthritis.
However, it gives temporary relief from the
physical or mental tension that always
makes pain worse. Nor can massage eliminate the cause of tension for those under
high levels of stress. But it relieves the
tension and combats feelings of isolation,
helping people feel better and cope more
effectively with stress.

Some adults have great difficulty relaxing, which takes a serious toll on their
bodies, personal relationships and quality of
life. This is the consequence of how they
learned to react to stress during childhood
and the cumulative amount of stress they
have experienced throughout life. They
tend to ignore their tension or mask it with
drugs and alcohol; this only allows more
tension to accumulate. My growing experi-

ence with massage led me to wonder if it could be used in a truly preventative fashion. Could massage during childhood teach relaxation skills at a deep level, preventing these huge accumulations of tension?

Over the years I also discovered, and became deeply concerned about, the fear of touch and intimacy in many adults, which caused isolation and loneliness. I wondered if massage could help by teaching children this warm, positive way to relate. Perhaps it could foster loving personal relationships so vital to physical and emotional health.

During my training as an infant massage teacher, I learned massage techniques and discovered the tremendous amount of research supporting the use of touch during infancy and childhood. Experts in many fields agree that touch is vital for healthy growth and development, and people of many cultures massage their babies and

children. For some cultures, such as China and India, massage has been a tradition for thousands of years.

When I began teaching infant massage, I was very pleased at the results. At the end of a five-week class, babies were more comfortable being massaged and relaxed much more deeply than before. Massage helped reduce crankiness, insomnia, and pain from gas and constipation. Parents found the massage time relaxing and fun. I began massaging my own children when they were a few weeks old. They were excellent models for classes, demonstrations in front of large groups and even on television, because they were so relaxed and happy while being massaged. As they've grown, I've done massage with them to also help them relax, help them sleep, and to relieve minor aches and pains. I've received additional training in massage for children with special needs, and worked with many of them. I am now thoroughly convinced that sensitive, caring massage is wonderful for children.

Massage has been effective in helping children learn to relax. With practice, even small children can let body tension dissolve when gently touched and urged to let go. A three-year-old girl, who heard the same piece of music every time her mother massaged her as a baby, now can relax just by listening to the music. As children release accumulated tension they feel happier and more relaxed, and often fall asleep. Childcare centers have found that back rubs are very helpful in slowing down active small children at naptime. (Relaxation training of any type—from yoga to biofeedback—teaches children to discriminate between different states of body arousal or tension and to have some control over their fight-or-flight response.) For parents too, massage is a wonderful excuse to set aside quiet time for relaxation.

Children love being massaged. They look forward to the quiet time and the special

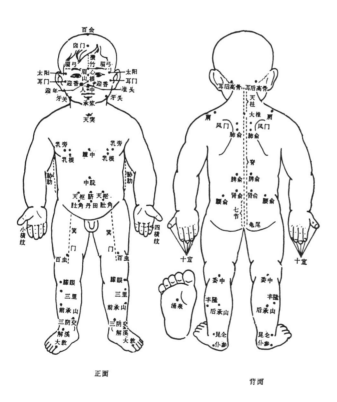

A diagram of tuina (Chinese medical massage) points, from Turtle Tail and Other Tender Mercies: Traditional Chinese Pediatrics *(Blue Poppy Press)*

attention from Mom or Dad, and ask to be massaged for aches and pains or insomnia, and when they are sick or insecure. They are very comfortable with touch, and even massage others—including their parents! Two-year-olds teach their friends how to massage, and older children give backrubs to young siblings who are hurt or tired.

Parents say they feel closer to their children by communicating through touch. When I massage my children, each of us grows more aware of the other's physical and emotional self. Massage provides us with a great deal of information and feedback about each other, for body language is truly the most intense and immediate form of communication. A mother who gives her two teenagers a backrub at bedtime tells me that this is the time when her children confide in her. Touch can help increase communication between parent and child

throughout life, enriching the relationship far beyond childhood. A middle-aged man told me that his elderly father has sounded increasingly senile over the phone. However, he says, "If I go back to see him, and I just sit and hold his hand long enough, after a while he doesn't sound so senile any more." Some American hospices teach massage techniques to families of the terminally ill; patients love receiving massages and their families are very happy to be able to do something so concrete, positive and loving for them.

Very few Americans are touched as much as they desire. Coping with tension and stress, as well as improving interpersonal relationships, are major concerns in our society today. I believe massage can be a small but significant step in addressing these concerns and providing families with more comfort, closeness and relaxation.

Acknowledgements

A great many people have contributed to the creation of this book. For critiquing the manuscript and offering moral support I must thank especially my personal literary lioness Naomi Krant; also Rebecca Taylor, Beth DeCamp, Sharon Gossman, and Kelly Tharp. The librarians at the Corvallis City Library and the Oregon State University Library were unfailingly helpful—and friendly to my children! Judy at Kinko's was also very nice to my kids, even when we practically lived there. Many thanks to all those who consented to be interviewed for the special needs chapter: Kathy Knowles, Pamela Yeaton, Meir Schneider, Helen Campbell, Marty Folin, Larry Burns-Vidlak, Deborah Bowes, Ann Perrault, and Kathleen Weber.

I truly appreciate Randy Fingland and Stan Nelson of Wingbow Press for their dedication to helping **Massage for Healthier Children** remain true to my original vision of it—and for being such nice people to work with.

Authors whose work has been especially informative and inspiring, and whose influence runs throughout these pages:

Christopher Lasch
Janet Travell
Hugh Drummond
David Werner
Agatha and Calvin Thrash
James Lynch
Meir Schneider.

Midwife Mabel Dzata has provided a shining example of what it means to care for someone's health.

Thanks to Diedrich Dasenbrock for the wonderful photographs which served as the source of Richard Robertson's drawings, and to all the parents and children who modelled for them.

Many thanks to those who have taught me the most about massage, and who have honored me by letting me share their lives—my clients.

I am deeply indebted to my husband Michael, whose support for my work has come in many forms, and without whom **Massage For Healthier Children** would never have been written. Finally I thank my wonderful children Rachel and Daniel, who have been teaching me since the day they were born, and make worthwhile the work of parenting.

Introduction

Massage is a wonderful gift for a parent to give a child. It warms, soothes, and communicates affection with a richness nothing else can match. It can also reduce muscular tension, relieve minor discomforts, and teach the ability to relax. Loving touch is like good nutrition, exercise, and adequate sleep—a simple but indispensable part of health and well-being. Eighteen years of practicing and teaching massage have convinced me that every parent can learn how to give an excellent massage by using the techniques presented here. All you need besides this book is lotion or massage oil, a few simple items you already have around the house, and quiet time with your child.

Chapter One discusses what massage can do for your child. Chapter Two tells you how to create a relaxing setting and what accessories you need, and discusses communication during massage. Chapter Three is a step-by-step guide to giving a complete massage to any child over the age of two. The strokes are easy, and the more you do them the easier they will become. Optional advanced techniques are also included. Chapter Four shows you how to massage away "minor" discomforts such as tension headaches, and Chapter Five discusses how to deal with problems you may encounter. Chapter Six shows you how massage can be used for children with special needs. Additional information can be found in four appendices, a bibliography, and a resource section.

Massage has many wonderful aspects. It is a satisfying handcraft, a vehicle for teaching relaxation, trust and body awareness, and a tangible expression of caring for others. **Massage For Healthier Children** has been written so that more families can discover the joys and benefits of massage. Laying-on of hands, including massage, has been a healing technique since the dawn of recorded history. I have seen it work for thousands of people, young and old. As you learn to massage your family, I am sure you will be pleasantly surprised at just how much comfort, closeness and relaxation your hands can bring.

One
The Value of Massage

I started doing massage with my kids to get more in tune with them, and then it turned into a fun thing to see how they responded. Nicole (9) will open up during massage and talk about things she wouldn't otherwise. She wants me to massage her a lot. She had a serious bicycle accident last year, which did a lot of damage to her front teeth, so I massaged her to help reduce the pain she had in her neck and upper back. I use massage with Valerie (6) to draw her out when she is sulky or not getting along with the rest of the family. Daniel (2) has Down's Syndrome, and I have done massage with him for a lot of reasons—to help him gain weight, help him relax, give him extra stimulation, and to help us bond.[1]

This chapter answers the question, "What is the value of massaging my child?" In it you will learn about the value of massage for the parent-child relationship. You will also learn about the nature of tension and stress in children, and how massage can relieve it. The benefits of massage are grouped into several categories. However, when you give or receive a mas-sage, the experience as a whole is much more than the sum of the parts. Comfort, closeness and relaxation happen together, affecting mind, emotions and body at the same time.

Comfort: Physical

A couple of years back I took care of a nine-year-old boy who had been a quadriplegic and on a respirator for five years. . . . He really enjoyed the massage. It gave him a lot of sensory stimulation as well as relaxation.[2]

Massage relieves excess muscular tension, stiffness and minor aches and pains, whether their cause is physical or emotional. As you feel the massaged area become softer, warmer and more pliant, your child will feel a melting away of soreness from strenuous exercise, tension headache or stomachache, muscular fatigue or stress-caused muscle spasm.

Here are some of the effects of massage that make it so valuable:
• It stretches muscle and connective tissue, relieving muscle spasm.

• It stimulates local circulation of both blood and lymphatic fluid. Constricted blood vessels dilate, and the blood supply to the massaged area increases, as much as tripling in five minutes. Your manual pressure moves lymphatic fluid out of the area; this hastens elimination of wastes and can significantly relieve swelling.

• Touch and massage encourage production of vital hormones. For example, several studies have found that premature babies who are massaged gain weight faster on the same amount of formula than those who are not, possibly because massage stimulates the production of somatotropin, a growth hormone.[3] Touch can also stimulate production of the painkilling hormone endorphin.[4]

Many parents use small massage treatments to help their children. They may massage a newborn baby's tear duct to unblock it. Rubbing tender gums in a teething baby relieves swelling that causes discomfort. Rubbing an injection site after an immunization keeps it from bruising. Vibrating or pounding the chest loosens mucus secretions in children with chronic respiratory diseases such as cystic fibrosis, or children recuperating from heart surgery. Massage relieves muscle cramps that occur in the leg at night. In addition, many parents instinctively rub their children's backs to help them relax or sleep.

As you massage your child and the muscles under your hands relax, other parts of the body become less tense. Stress not only causes contraction of skeletal muscles (such as those of the face, back and legs), but also of muscles lining internal organs (including arteries, lungs, stomach and intestines). As your child enters a state of deep relaxation, all these contracted muscles let go. In our culture, which emphasizes appearance and performance under pressure over relaxation and comfort, some children might never otherwise have this experience.

Comfort: Emotional

Caring human touch has an extraordinary power to soothe, reassure, and relieve anxiety. While working in a hospital emergency room, I noticed that many nurses and doctors instinctively held the hands of frightened patients, gently touched those with severe pain, or put an arm around the shoulders of hysterical ones. Patients deeply appreciated sensitive touch in this stressful situation. On the other hand, some health workers stayed distant; I observed one doctor listening to a patient's heart with one hand on his stethoscope and the other in his pocket, not making contact with either hand. Patients treated in this distant way felt more anxious, more isolated and less cared

SYLVIA   **by Nicole Hollander**

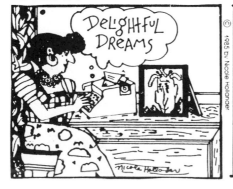

for. A study at the Royal Edinburgh Hospital investigated the use of massage to treat patients with a history of severe anxiety and difficulty relaxing. They received sessions of back massage; at the same time, they were taken off all anti-anxiety drugs. As a result of the massage treatments, some patients significantly reduced their dosage of drugs, while others discontinued them altogether.[5] Similar results were found with teenagers in a hospital psychiatric ward.[6]

In *Touching and Being Touched*, Robert Coles describes the power of touch to provide comfort and stability. He witnessed the courage of black children and their parents during the struggle for school integration in New Orleans in 1961. He was profoundly moved by the strength the young students showed as they faced white mobs. A mother of one of the children described her daughter's response to the school day:

My child comes home from school, and she's heard those white people shouting, and she's not going to show them she's scared, not for a second, but she is scared, I know she is. And the first thing she does is come to me, and I hold her. Then she goes get her snack, the Oreos and juice, and she's back touching me. I'll be upset myself, so thank God my mother is still with us, because I go to her, and she'll put her hand on my arm, and I'm all settled down again, and then I can put my hand on my daughter's arm! Like our minister says, the Lord touches us all the time, if we'll just let Him, and He works through each of us, so when my mother puts her hands on me, and I put my hands on my child—it's God giving us strength.[7]

Massage is a wonderful extension of the natural impulse to communicate love and concern through touch. Most parents do this instinctively when their children are troubled; massage, however, adds much more.

Closeness

Caring touch is an important part of every intimate relationship; to make physical contact is to make emotional contact. Touch between parents and children communicates caring, builds trust, and affirms our biological connection. Babies and children differ in their individual response to touch, but all appear to need and enjoy it. Children who are deprived of tactile stimulation often shy away from touch, although they really crave it. They are much more likely to become violent adults than children who were given lots of physical affection. For these children, loving touch is powerful and effective therapy. Psychotherapists have used holding, massage and other forms of body contact to fulfill the need for touch and closeness, and to build trust.

Baby animals have been found to produce endorphins (sedative-like chemicals manufactured by the brain with a chemical structure similar to many narcotics) when in touch with their mothers. This suggests that touch deprivation and loneliness may be linked with drug abuse. According to psychologist Sidney Jourard, extensive physical contact may be a primordial sedative and tranquilizer. "I see sedatives as encapsulated caresses and massage... The lonely, who lack a lover to caress them to sleep, turn to barbiturates."[8]

It is terribly sad to see an adult lying on a massage table full of apprehension at the prospect of being touched. This fearful adult may have grown up in a non-touching family, or suffered physical trauma, painful medical treatment, or even physical or sexual abuse. When this happens, a child may learn to deny the need for touch, and avoid it altogether; as a result, what starts as a survival strategy leads to touch deprivation and social isolation with few strong friendships. Besides being very painful, isolation is extremely detrimental to health;

living a life cut off from others significantly increases one's chance of dying prematurely.[9] Before massage can relieve muscle tension or teach relaxation skills, a touch-phobic person must learn to tolerate touch itself. With gentle, sensitive touch over a period of time, trust can be built, fear of touch decreased, and the benefits of massage obtained.

Relaxation

When I started pediatric practice in 1933, parents worried about polio and pneumonia and ear abscesses. Now they worry about drugs and teenage pregnancy and nuclear annihilation.
—*Benjamin Spock*[10]

Today's children undergo stresses radically different from those of yesterday. However, it would be unrealistic to romanticize the past, when there was a great deal more physical suffering. Until about two hundred years ago, three quarters of all children died before the age of five, chiefly of infectious diseases. Children were also expected to begin hard physical labor at an early age, and child abuse and exploitation were common. During the Middle Ages, children of six or seven were believed capable of working like adults and being exposed to adult matters such as sexuality and death.

Around the end of the eighteenth century, Western society saw the rise of a new attitude toward children; childhood was considered a special stage in life, with attributes such as innocence, imagination, and closeness to nature. Parents struggled to preserve their children's innocence, shelter them from life's ups and downs, and keep childhood a carefree "golden age." In our time, modern medicine and such public health measures as clean drinking water and pasteurization of milk have greatly reduced childhood illness and mortality rates. Children are no longer expected to perform adult physical labor.

Life should now be much easier for our children. But physical stress has been superseded by psychological stress. Social changes have caused parents to change the way they think about childhood. Increasing

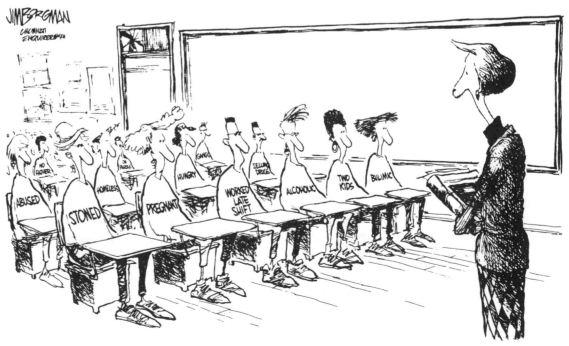

GOOD MORNING, TEACHER

numbers of parents now believe that children should have an adult understanding of reality, preparing them to survive an increasingly complex and uncontrollable world. However, exposing children to adult realities before they are developmentally mature enough to handle them can be highly stressful. Economic changes also play a part; for example, in many of today's families, both parents work and children are often left unsupervised, making childhood innocence much more difficult to preserve.

Q. Do the new stresses on kids make them better equipped to deal with adult stresses? A. No. Human beings do make some adjustment to stresses, but that doesn't mean that they're doing better by being brought up with stresses. It's going to make them more tense, more harsh, more intensely competitive, and more greedy.—Benjamin Spock[11]

Consider the new, primarily psychological stresses affecting children today:
• Vastly greater exposure to the adult world's problems at earlier ages than ever before through the mass media, especially television. Watching TV also precludes pure play, one of the best ways for children to truly relax.
• Deterioration of family support: The amount of time parents spend with their children dropped 40 percent between 1965 and 1989.[12]
• Divorce rates continue to climb, and the help available from the extended family continues to decline.
• High incidence of physical and sexual abuse.
• Loss of religious beliefs and the support of religious communities.
• Severely competitive conditions beginning as early as kindergarten, decreasing time spent in play.
• Inadequate childcare, followed by schools which fail to educate or provide for personal identity needs.

• Poverty, perhaps the greatest stressor of all. In America today one out of five children is poor and likely to be in a single-parent family. A child growing up in poverty is more apt to experience abuse, neglect, malnutrition, ill health, homelessness, and substandard day care. Childhood poverty also places young people at risk for a range of longterm problems, including poor health, failure in school, teenage pregnancy, crime and drug abuse.

What is the evidence that these new and more powerful stresses are taking a toll on children?
• Increasingly widespread school dropout rates, juvenile crime, substance abuse, severe depression and suicide.
• Sexual activity beginning at younger ages, with attendant risks of pregnancy and venereal disease, including AIDS.
• Type A behavior as a way of coping with stress, characterized by competitiveness, impatience, restlessness and aggression. Type A behavior is considered a major risk factor in the development of heart disease. (See Appendix C, page 83.)
• Hyperactive behavior. Prescription of the drug Ritalin to treat hyperactivity increased sixfold between 1971 and 1989. Many child psychologists and medical professionals believe Ritalin is increasingly prescribed for children whose hyperactive behavior is caused by stress.[13] Relaxation training and massage are effective in reducing this type of "hyperactivity", whereas Ritalin only suppresses symptoms.
• Psychosomatic illness. As many as 35 percent of American children suffer stress-related health problems at some point.[14]

Of course, we cannot turn the clock back to an earlier time. We need to recognize the stresses that affect our children, then look for ways to reduce stress where possible, and teach children to cope. Massage and relaxation training are among the most effective and easily available methods of doing this.

Children's Response to Stress

Although children encounter different types of stress than adults, their physiological response to it is the same. In what is known as the "fight-or-flight response," the body's different systems gear up in a variety of ways.

• The adrenal glands release the anti-inflammatory hormone cortisone. Continued high levels of cortisone hamper the ability to fight off both major and minor illnesses, and may also lead to stomach ulcers.

• The thyroid gland secretes thyroxin, a hormone which speeds up the body's metabolism. Excess thyroxin can lead to shaky nerves, insomnia, and exhaustion.

• Endorphin, a painkilling hormone, is released in greater amounts by the brain. Eventually, endorphin supplies are depleted and pain tolerance decreases.

• Shutdown of secretion and movement in the digestive tract diverts blood to the skeletal muscles. Continued shutdown can lead to digestive discomfort such as cramps, nausea, bloating, and diarrhea.

• The level of sugar in the blood rises, and the pancreas produces more insulin to metabolize it. Chronic elevation can accustom one to crave sugar. Diabetes can be started or aggravated by excessive demands on the pancreas to produce insulin.

• Cholesterol flows from the liver into the bloodstream. Sustained high levels can cause deposits of cholesterol to accumulate in the blood vessels, leading to arteriosclerosis and heart disease.

• The heart beats harder and faster. On a long-term basis, this can lead to high blood pressure, increasing the risk of stroke and heart attack.

• All five senses become more acute. Excessive stress, over time, will eventually cause the senses to be exhausted, and less efficient. Ability to concentrate is greatly decreased.

• Muscle tension increases, resulting in feelings of tension and stiffness, decreased freedom of movement, and sometimes pain such as headache or stomachaches. The individual finds it increasingly difficult to relax when not under stress.

In more primitive times the fight-or-flight response was a vitally necessary means of survival. But in today's world of psychological stresses, the ability to induce a relaxation response is crucial.

A child who cannot relax suffers a buildup of tension that can become crushing. The child's muscles, both skeletal and internal, may be tensed or braced at all times, expending tremendous energy. Some very tense children are constantly restless, and look and feel tight inside and out. Their outer muscles feel knotted and hard. Other children react to tension in another way; they look tired, act hopeless, and feel limp inside. Their bodies may feel soft at first touch, but there is great tension in the deeper skeletal muscles and those of the stomach, intestines, and eyes. In both cases, emotional and physical fatigue interfere with body comfort, the ability to concentrate and the individual's sense of control.

Excessive stress, causing the reactions discussed above, plays a part in numerous illnesses. One recent medical book mentions twenty-six stress-related conditions, ranging from tension headaches and high blood pressure, to ulcers and back pain.[15] These stress-related problems can affect children from infancy through adolescence. A 1973 study examined the relationship between stress and illness in families with children under the age of eighteen. Mothers recorded upsetting events and illness in their families over a month. Researchers found that the chance of developing fevers, colds, or other minor illness after a stressful event increased 50 percent for children and doubled for mothers.[16] Other studies have shown that children with major physical illnesses, prior to the onset of their illness, have experienced twice the stress of control populations of healthy children.[17]

Another reaction to physical or emotional trauma in a specific body area is a habit of always tensing that area when stressed. Examples of traumas include injuries, severe burns, surgery, and sexual or physical abuse. Fear of having the area retraumatized causes muscles in the area to contract, creating a shield or wall. Muscular shielding is an instinctual survival mechanism that may be useful immediately after injury to prevent blood loss or harmful movement of a hurt area. But it is detrimental when the area becomes chronically tense out of habit.

Muscular shielding can begin very early in life. For example, if blood samples are taken from a baby's feet over a long period, the baby's feet may become very tense and "touchy." According to a nurse who works in a neonatal intensive care unit, the babies there get to know who takes blood samples, and they tense their legs and feet when that person arrives. Another example is a baby who was pricked in the neck by a needle when his mother had amniocentesis in her eighth month of pregnancy. At sixteen months of age he had such a severe neck spasm that his head was pinned to one shoulder and he could barely crawl. He had contracted his neck muscles before birth and never relaxed them![18]

In recent years children have shown that they can increase their body awareness and control their muscle tension through biofeedback, visual imagery, yoga, and relaxation of different muscle groups. Using these techniques they can cope with mental problems such as learning disabilities and hyperactivity, emotional problems such as phobias and test anxiety, and physical problems such as tension headaches, asthma and burn pain.

Massage is deeply relaxing, especially when combined with simple relaxation techniques. As a massage progresses and the receiver lets go of tension, external signs of relaxation can be seen. Breathing becomes slower and deeper, and skin becomes pinker and warmer. Faces soften, hands and feet unclench, and the whole body sinks into the massage table. Occasionally people cry

while releasing particularly deep tension. Researchers have found significant internal changes as well. Blood chemistry, heartrate, blood pressure, muscle fiber length, and the circulation of blood and lymph are altered. Measurements of these functions have shown that even children in comas respond to gentle touch.[19]

Massage is also an excellent way to change the tendency to shield a traumatized area by contracting it. Mothers whose babies have tension in their feet from blood sampling can teach their babies to relax again, using gentle massage and relaxation exercises done at the babies' pace. Older children with tension or guarding around old injuries can learn to relax those areas. Adults have much more difficulty learning new patterns, because the old ones are so ingrained. How much simpler and easier to massage children whose habits are not already established!

Sometimes long-forgotten childhood memories return during a state of deep relaxation. Severe local muscle tension can occur when troubling emotions or experiences are unresolved; as the tension begins to ease, the original trauma is recalled, and the emotion accompanying it released. I have seen massage trigger recollections of physical and sexual abuse, painful emotional experiences, and traumatic injuries.

By using the massage and relaxation techniques in this book, you can help your child cope with stress and accumulated tension in a number of important ways:

You will teach your child how to recognize and control tension before it becomes overwhelming.

You can prevent chronic muscular shielding in areas that have been traumatized.

You will provide a positive role model, demonstrating both self-help skills and concern for your child's welfare.

In addition, if you use the relaxation techniques as you massage your child, massage time will be relaxing and educational for you as well.

TWO
Before You Begin

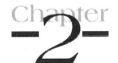

When receiving a good massage a person usually falls into a mental-physical state difficult to describe. It is like entering a special room until now locked and hidden away; a room the very existence of which is likely to be familiar only to those who practice some form of daily meditation.—George Downing, The Massage Book[1]

In Chapter One you learned about the beneficial effects of massage. In this chapter you will learn how to prepare for a massage. Read this chapter once, carefully. Then, before you begin massaging, look over the checklist on page 12 to make sure you have everything you need.

The first step is to create the right environment for massage, where your child feels warm, comfortable and secure, and you can relax and concentrate. There may be times when your child needs a little massage, but you can't go off by yourselves or don't want to go to the trouble of setting up a massage environment. It's fine to grab a towel and a bottle of lotion or oil, and have your child flop down on the sofa, the lawn, or on the floor in front of the TV. First, however, you should practice the massage strokes in Chapter Four in a quiet, unhurried setting so that you're familiar with them and can give your child the massage she needs, wherever you are.

What You Bring: Communication and Attitude

When I was a medical student and my first child was nearly five, he complained so severely about a belly ache that I was worried he might have appendicitis. I asked him to lie down on his bed and sat beside him to examine his belly. As I laid my hand on him to begin to press, he screamed with pain. I asked him if his belly was really that tender, and he said, with tears in his eyes, "No, no, you're sitting on my foot!" —Mary Howell, Healing at Home[2]

Clear communication during massage helps your child relax, helps you give a massage that meets your child's needs, and increases your sensitivity to each

9

other. Successful communication is both verbal and non-verbal. It's also important to consider how your attitude affects your massage.

Verbal Communication

Feedback is important while you are learning massage, so you know how much pressure to use, which strokes feel best, and so on. Because it is difficult to talk and relax at the same time, the majority of the massage should be done quietly. But be sure to ask your child how the strokes feel.

Also, because comfort is essential, make it clear that you want to know if something hurts or tickles, if the room is too cold, if any area feels particularly sore or sensitive, or if your child has had enough massage. Do not massage any area your child does not want touched. Always ask, if you are in doubt. When your child knows that his or her needs will be respected, then it is much easier to relax.

In general, use positive phrases such as "relax deeply," rather than negative ones such as "don't tense up." Be sure to give your child lots of positive reinforcement whenever you see signs of relaxation. If you see tensing and holding on, communicate this in a gentle, non-critical way. Then say something like "Okay, can you let your hand just rest in mine?" or "Now take a deep breath and relax a little more." Refer to the basic relaxation sequence on page 15 for other suggestions. If your child loosens up even a tiny bit, give lots of praise. The longer I practice massage, the more respect I have for the self-healing restorative powers of the human body; I like to communicate this to the person receiving the massage. I acknowledge that even though he or she may be experiencing discomfort or tension, there are countless ways in which his or her body is functioning very

well. I may point some of these out, such as the ability to move, heal from injuries, digest food, and so on.

Non-Verbal Communication: What Your Hands Say

Your hands express your moods and feelings by how tight or soft they are, how abruptly or gently you put them on your child, and how fast or slowly you move them. When you are tense, you are more likely to hold your hands stiffly, put them on your child in a sudden, invasive way, or massage too jerkily or too fast. If you feel tense, help yourself and your child by consciously relaxing and slowing down. Do the basic relaxation sequence together if necessary.

If your pressure is causing pain or flinching, regardless of what the massage instructions say, lighten your pressure or move on to another area. If you cause pain because you want to do the massage a certain way, you indicate that your child's feelings are unimportant. Sore, tight or traumatized areas need a gentle touch. Too much pressure may actually cause more tension, or give the message that "pain is good for you." Gently touching your child communicates your affection and respect for him or her as an individual.

What Your Hands Perceive During Massage

Physical tension. Tight muscles feel thicker, more bunched up and sometimes colder than relaxed muscles. When you first touch them, they do not give with your pressure. As muscles relax, you will feel them soften and become warmer. When an area of the body is tense, you will also feel that it is tightly fixed, and once the area is relaxed you'll feel less rigidity there. For example, if the chest, back and abdominal muscles are very tight, the ribs are pinned down; expansion of the ribcage during inhalation is impossible and breathing is shallow. When the muscles are relaxed after massage, the ribs are less restricted and during inhalation the whole chest can expand much more.

Emotional tension. Your child flinches or withdraws from your hands. You may feel your child tensing another part of the body, gasping, breathing fast or not at all. Many children and adults in our culture have learned to hide their tension, even from themselves, but with practice your hands will sense subtle signs. The more massage you do, the more sensitive to body language you will become. This will help you relate more closely, understand how your child is dealing with stress, and give you more empathy for your child.

Communicating Your Attitude

When I am doing massage, whether with an adult or a child, my first priority is to help him or her relax as deeply as possible; everything I do is directed towards this goal. It often requires persistance, ingenuity and respect for individual differences. Here are some important points I keep in mind as I work:

Put the individual's needs first. If the person needs to talk, I encourage that, although I want him or her to eventually take advantage of the peace and quiet for real relaxation. If the person cannot relax while nude, the clothes stay on and we do relaxation exercises and pressure point massage. If he or she doesn't want certain parts of the body touched, I don't touch them.

It is not a good idea to use massage to meet your own agenda. For example, when my daughter was two I tried to use massage to get her to sleep, although she wasn't the sleepy one; I was, and I wanted a break! Another example would be using massage to pin a child down to discuss a conflict-ridden topic, such as grades or chores.

Be comfortable yourself. If you have not had a touch-oriented relationship with your child and you are trying to create one, go slowly and do just a little massage at first. If you feel truly uncomfortable about touching your child, don't do it! I recommend that you talk about your discomfort with a trusted friend, a professional counselor, or someone whose profession involves a lot of touching. It is surprising how common discomfort with touch is; it usually stems from a negative experience such as physical pain or trauma, physical or sexual abuse, or lack of touch in the formative years. An anorexic woman once brought her child to one of my infant massage classes to help him form a positive image of his body. She had not been touched at all during her childhood and realized this was one reason she had such problems with her own body image. She hardly knew how to touch her son at all. I recommended she receive some massage herself to help her learn what caring touch felt like; this would be the first step in learning how to touch sensitively.

If you feel angry or upset with your child, don't do massage; your feelings will come right through your hands, and very likely neither of you will feel relaxed. If you feel drained or exhausted, take care of yourself by getting some rest or relaxation.

What You Will Need

Quiet Time. Quiet surroundings and freedom from interruption are ideal. Distractions make it more difficult for your child to relax deeply. Plan to spend at least fifteen to twenty minutes. (You will probably need longer when you're first learning.) Bedtime is usually best, not only because this is already a quiet time for your child, but because massage promotes deep restful sleep. Also, when you first introduce massage to an active small child, this may be the only time he or she will settle down! Once you have learned the technique, you may want to tell your child a soothing bedtime story while you massage.

Warmth. Wherever you are doing massage should be at least 70 degrees if your child has removed most of his or her clothes. Keep a sheet or towel on hand in case of chills. If you are doing a partial massage, only the area being massaged needs to be uncovered, so the room can be somewhat cooler. A hot bath or shower is an excellent way to warm up and relax before a massage. Small children can even be massaged in the bathtub, using soap instead of oil.

Soft Lighting. Glaring lights cause eye tension and give a room a harsh feeling. Soft, indirect lighting or natural light is best.

Massage Oil or Lotion. Natural oils such as safflower or almond are ideal, and can be bought in any supermarket or health food store. Ordinary skin lotion also works, but must be applied more often as it soaks into the skin. If you are doing massage at bedtime and your child will go right to sleep, lotion is preferable because it leaves the skin less oily. Keep oils and lotions in squeeze bottles (such as old shampoo bottles) that won't spill if you knock them over. It's easy to warm oil or lotion by setting the bottle in a bowl of hot water.

Massage Surface. If you are doing just one or two parts of the body, use your child's bed. If you are doing more, use your dining room table or floor. The surface must be soft and comfortable. Cover with padding and a sheet.

Linens. Start with padding for the table or floor. Use a few thick blankets or folded-out sleeping bags, or a foam pad. Cover the bed or padding with a sheet or towel. This will keep oil from soaking through. Put a pillow or rolled-up towel under knees or ankles.

Your Hands. The most important ingredient of all. Wash them and remove all rings, watches, and bracelets. Long nails scratch and hurt the skin, so clip them before you begin.

Now you know what to bring, and in the next chapter, you'll learn what to do.

Checklist

✓ Quiet time
✓ Warmth—room temperature 70 degrees or more
✓ Soft lighting
✓ Massage oil or lotion in a squeeze bottle
✓ Massage surface, padded and covered
✓ Linens: padding if using table or floor, two sheets or towels, and one pillow or rolled-up towel
✓ Your hands—washed, with short nails and no jewelry

Three
A Full Body Massage

For maybe 4 or 5 months bedtime had been one of the most unpleasant times of the day. At least 1—1½ hours of arguments and squabbles lay before us. It was primed by a buildup of energy with no place to go, coming right up against the time to relax and sleep. I felt disappointed, defeated, and angry and each night my patience grew thinner. "A massage," I said, "with oil!" Finn (6½) and Madigan (4) loved the idea. It would be a challenge as I would have to massage them together: first one back, then the other and so on... It would be nice to be able to set a calm mood, but the massage begins with wild energy and ends with a yawn—in between there are squabbles: "When's it my turn?"—"Madigan's on my side of the bed!" Even so, the moment my hands touch a little boy's back, everything feels solid, matter of fact, and yet not without feeling. By the end of the massage, everything is quiet (relatively) and the breathing deeper.
—Barbara Haley, quoted in Tender Loving Care[1]

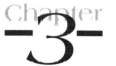

So far you have learned why to massage, what essentials you need, and about communication during massage. In this chapter, you will learn *how* to do massage.

The Massage Technique

The technique you will learn is a modified form of Swedish/Esalen massage. It is gentle and slow-paced, and incorporates relaxation for both child and parent. Massage of each part of the body begins with a simple relaxation exercise. Then the first massage stroke gently warms the entire area, introducing touch in a relaxing and non-threatening way. The following strokes release tension in smaller, more specific areas. The first stroke is repeated often to remind the entire area to stay relaxed. You'll finish massaging each area with this stroke as well, and conclude with the relaxation exercise.

Doing every stroke in this chapter in order would take about forty-five minutes. With small children who move around a lot, each part of the body may take less time. If you wish to massage just one part of the body, set aside at least fifteen to twenty minutes. Never rush through a massage. You do not need to do the parts of the body in the order presented here, but never begin on an area that feels especially vulnerable to your child, such as a ticklish area or the site of an old injury.

How to Learn the Massage Strokes

Begin by reading the section called "Basic Techniques" (page 15). While you are learning, massage only one part of the body each time. Begin by reading the instructions for that part twice. Now position yourself comfortably with the book open in front of you; if you are in an uncomfortable position, you'll be more tense and easily fatigued. Go through the relaxation sequence, apply oil, and practice each stroke, referring to the book as needed.

Take plenty of breaks at first so you do not become overtired. The first few times you practice, it will take you longer to do the strokes and you may feel clumsy or awkward. Persevere—your child will love your massage even if it's not perfect! Remember, the loving relationship that you and your child share puts you far ahead of the world's most expert massage therapist. After a little practice, you will feel much more confident and smooth. Be sure to ask for feedback from your child. After you have learned the strokes, you may tear out or copy the full body massage checklist (page 110) and put it on the wall, referring to it rather than the book.

Adapting Massage to Your Child

Because every child is a unique individual, you may need to alter your massage rather than trying to do exactly what is outlined here. Your child can generally tell you what best suits him or her, but here are some general guidelines, based on interviews with numerous parents.

Attention span. Children are truly individuals when it comes to how long they will lie quietly while you massage them. Younger children usually have a shorter attention span, although this is not always true; some toddlers will lie still for a full body massage while some older children will relax for only five minutes.

For children who can't seem to lie still, you have to be flexible and try different solutions.
• Use soap and massage your child's upper body while he or she is in the bathtub.
• Massage at naptime or bedtime when your child is tired.
• Follow your child around as he or she plays. One mother says she can massage her two-year-old son this way forever, "as long as I don't interfere with his play."
• One resourceful mother found that if she put a hot towel, fresh from the dryer, under her daughter, she would lie still much longer.
• Massage your toddler's legs during a diaper change.
• Telling a story or singing may occupy a small child. When my daughter was less than two, I sang endless rounds of "Old MacDonald Had a Farm," gave her books and toys, and even let her smear lotion on my face as I massaged hers.
• Remember that the amount of time you massage your child is not as important as the fact that your child will know that he or she can ask you for a massage whenever desired.

Amount of pressure. This can vary from day to day, but most children usually prefer a certain type of pressure. Preferences range from extremely light to very firm. Some children ask for firmer pressure over very tight areas, or light pressure over sore areas.

The best area to massage. When in doubt, massage the back. Avoid any areas where your child doesn't like to be massaged or which cause discomfort. Children will often request certain areas such as the back for relaxation, insomnia and shoulder tension; the stomach for stomachaches; the face for relaxation; the legs for insomnia or growing pains; the neck for tension headaches; the feet for fatigue or discomfort following vigorous exercise.

Which strokes to use. Do more strokes your child enjoys, and fewer (or none) of the strokes he or she doesn't like. When in doubt, use smooth, even warming strokes. One mother says that her eleven-year-old son only likes warming strokes, and giggles and flinches when she does anything else. So every night she uses only the warming strokes for his back and legs, and both mother and child relax and enjoy the massage.

When Not to Massage

Do not massage skin that has sores, cuts, burns, boils or infectious rashes such as scabies. Do not massage inflamed joints, tumors, or any undiagnosed lumps. In the event of injuries (such as severe bruises, joint sprains, broken bones or dislocations) or medical conditions, consult with your doctor before you begin massage.

Basic Techniques: Applying Oil or Lotion

Your hands should be clean. Warm them by rubbing your palms together. Pour a small amount of oil or lotion into a cupped palm and let it warm in your hands. Use enough so your hands can slide easily but there is still some friction. More lotion can be applied occasionally. Gently smooth it over the entire area you will be massaging.

The Basic Relaxation Sequence

Each time you begin to massage a new part of the body, practice this simple relaxation sequence. It is very simple, takes a short time, and yields profound results. It greatly enhances the relaxing effect of the massage and teaches both of you a skill you can use anywhere, anytime. The more you practice it, the more deeply you'll be able to relax.

Both you and your child should take a few deep, comfortable breaths. As you exhale, consciously relax. Drop your shoulders, allow your face to soften, and relax your hands. If you feel tight anyplace, let go of tension there as you exhale. Suggest ways for your child to relax while exhaling, such as:

"Feel your stomach get nice and soft."

"Let your shoulders melt like ice."

"Let your muscles melt like butter in the sun."

"Make believe you're going to sleep."

"Let your hands hang loose."

"Let your whole body relax and sink into the bed."

Praise your child whenever you see that he or she is relaxing.

Repeat this sequence when you finish massaging each part of the body.

Massage Strokes

Warming. This introductory stroke warms and relaxes each area you will be massaging. With your palms and fingertips touching your child, glide smoothly over the whole area and back again. Let your hands flow gently over the body contours. Use gentle pressure at first, as you help the entire area

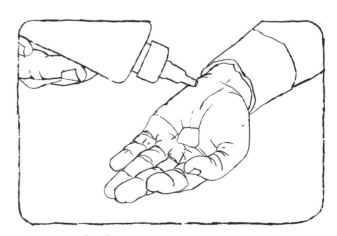

Warming oil or lotion.

become accustomed to your touch. After it is thoroughly warmed up, you may increase the pressure if it feels good to your child.

Raking. For the back, arms and legs, raking works on deeper tension. Curve and stiffen your fingers so your hand looks like a garden rake. (Did you clip your nails?) Begin at the top of the back or limb; use medium pressure. Drag the fingertips of one hand a short distance downward, then do the same with the fingertips of the other hand. Let your "rakes" overlap and work gradually down to the bottom of the area.

Kneading. This stroke, which stretches and relaxes large fleshy areas, is just like kneading bread dough. Use medium pressure; do not pinch, but squeeze gently. Grasp and lift a handful of flesh between the thumb and fingers of one hand. Slowly release as the other hand grasps the same tissue; lift and release it in turn. Continue alternating your hands.

Thumbstroking. This stroke covers smaller areas slowly and thoroughly. Use medium to firm pressure. Push away from you, first with the flat of one thumb and then with the other. Let these small pushes or strokes overlap slightly, and move in the direction specified.

An important note about optional variations: The variations are not part of the basic massage. They will be covered later as advanced technique (page 36); do not attempt to learn them now.

The Back

The back is a complex of muscles that work continuously during the day. Muscles of the arms, legs, neck and torso attach to the back and interweave with its complex musculature. By massaging the back, you release tension from all these areas. For this reason, if you can massage only one part of

the body, do the back. It's also a good place to begin a full body massage because most children feel comfortable about having their backs touched.

Have your child lie face down, arms at his or her side. Place a small rolled-up towel or pillow underneath the ankles. Sit on the side of the bed near your child's waistline.

Basic relaxation sequence (see page 15).

Apply oil or lotion.

Back warmer. Use gentle pressure. Begin by putting your hands down on the lower back. With hands parallel on either side of the spine, and your fingertips pointing toward the head, begin to glide towards the head. Move up the middle of the back, in between the shoulder blades, and up to the base of the neck. Now your hands will separate and glide out to the tip of each shoulder, down the sides of the torso and hips to the bottom of the buttocks, and return to starting position. Each hand is actually describing a large oval shape. Practice until this feels like one long stroke. Do ten times.
Optional variations:
Move up the back very slowly while pressing firmly just to either side of the spine.
Move up the back quickly and lightly, then move down the sides of the torso slowly and firmly.

Raking the back. Beginning at the shoulders, rake downwards. Use medium pressure. Each raking stroke should be an inch or two on a small child, and up to five or six inches on a teenager. Gradually move down one side of the back from the shoulders to the bottom of the buttocks. Now repeat on the other side. Repeat the whole stroke three times.

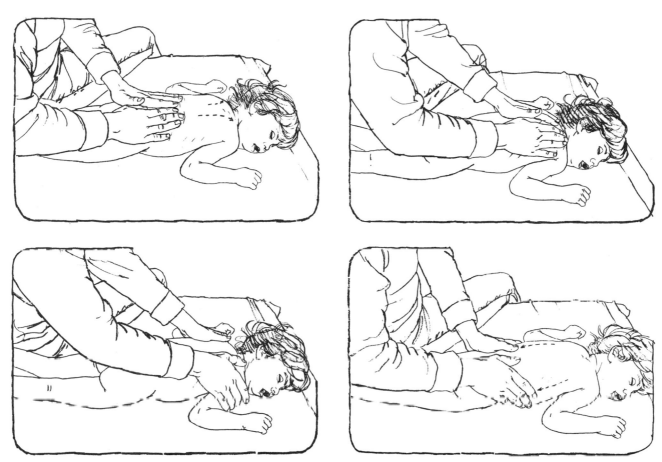

Back warmer.

Optional variations:

Vary your pressure from light to firm to light again.

Rake with your fingers farther apart or closer together.

Outline the inner edge of the shoulder blade with your fingertips, using tiny raking strokes as you move down.

Outline the back of the hipbone with your fingertips, using tiny raking strokes.

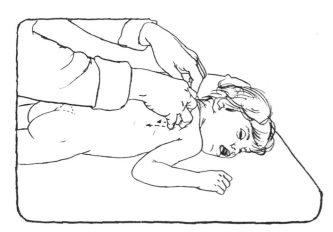

Raking the back.

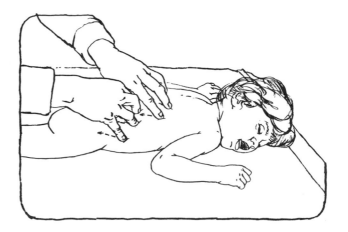

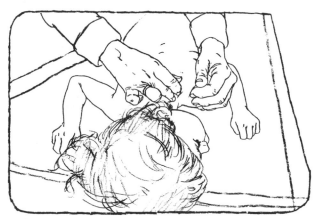

Kneading the shoulders.

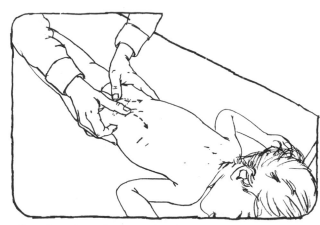

Thumbstroking the lower back.

Back warmer. Do three times.

Kneading the shoulders. Knead the muscles along the top of the shoulder, between the base of the neck and the tip of the shoulder. Use medium pressure. Do each side for thirty seconds or longer.
Back warmer. Do three times.

Thumbstroking the lower back. Just below the waistline, the back of the hipbone curves around and meets the sacrum, a triangular-shaped bone at the bottom of the spine. Beginning at the sacrum, use both thumbs to outline one hipbone at a time. Use medium to firm pressure. Push away from you, first with the flat of one thumb and then with the other. Let these small pushes

or strokes overlap slightly, and gradually slide out along the bone, all the way out to the side of the buttock. Imagine that you can define its shape with your thumbs. Do one whole side and repeat on the other, then use thumbstroke directly on top of the sacrum. Do once, slowly and thoroughly, taking approximately one minute. Note: This stroke can help relieve low back pain from strenuous exercise or tension.

Optional variations:
Vary the length of each push or stroke.
Use different speeds, from slow to fast.
Apply a variety of pressures, firm to light.

Kneading the buttocks. Knead the buttock muscles from the sacrum out to the side of the hip. Do one buttock, then the other. Use medium pressure. Do each buttock for thirty seconds or more. Note: This stroke can help relieve lower back pain resulting from strenuous exercise or tension.

Back warmer. Do three times.

Thumbstroking between the shoulder blades (not pictured). Work on the muscles between the shoulder blades, which are often very tense. Make short vertical pushes towards the head. Press firmly, but do not cause pain; if the area hurts, lighten your

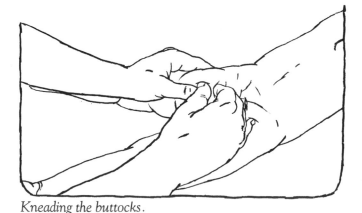

Kneading the buttocks.

pressure. Do for one minute or longer. Do not massage the spine itself.
Back warmer. Do ten times.

Basic relaxation sequence.

Back Massage Checklist

✓ Basic relaxation sequence.
✓ Apply oil or lotion.
✓ Back warmer ten times.
✓ Raking the back three times.
✓ Back warmer three times.
✓ Kneading the shoulders one minute.
✓ Back warmer three times.
✓ Thumbstroking the lower back one minute.
✓ Kneading the buttocks one minute.
✓ Back warmer three times.
✓ Thumbstroking between the shoulder blades one minute.
✓ Back warmer ten times.
✓ Basic relaxation sequence.

The Back of the Leg

Sit at the foot of the bed, near the outside of the child's foot. Small children may lay the entire leg across your lap.

Basic relaxation sequence (see page 15).

Apply oil or lotion.

Leg warmer. Use medium pressure. Place both palms on the ankle. With fingertips pointing towards the head and hands parallel, glide up to the top of the leg. Your inside hand will cover the inside of the leg and your outside hand will cover the outside portion. When you reach the top of the

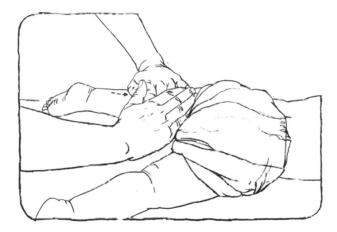

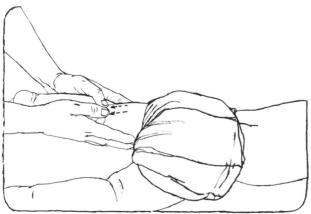

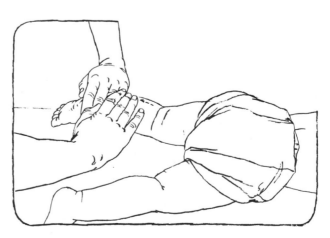

Leg warmer.

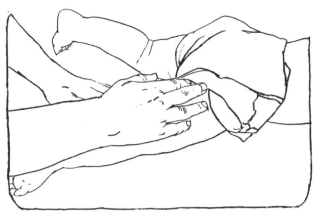

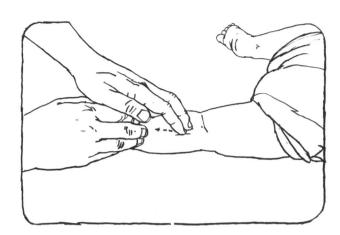

Raking the back of the leg.

leg, simply glide back down, again with your hands parallel. When you reach the foot, keep going and very gently stroke over the sole of the foot with your fingertips. Do not press on the back of the knee. Use gentle pressure for the entire stroke. Do ten times.

Raking the back of the leg. Sit opposite the back of the knee. Begin raking at the top of the buttock and work down to the back of the knee. Cover the muscles of the inner thigh, top of the thigh, and outside of the thigh. Do not press on the back of the knee itself. Now return to your original position at the foot of the bed and continue raking from the top of the calf to the ankle. Do the whole stroke—raking from buttock to ankle—once, using medium pressure. Go

slowly, so it takes one minute to rake the entire area once.

Optional variation: Vary the amount of pressure from medium to light; move very slowly.

Leg warmer three times.

Thumbstroking the sole of the foot. Begin at the base of the toes. Stroking away from you with your thumbs, work slowly and thoroughly up to the heel. Imagine that your thumbs are dipped in ink and you want to completely ink the entire sole. This is an area where firm pressure often feels good; ask your child what pressure is best. Do once, slowly, so that thumbstroking the entire sole takes a full minute.

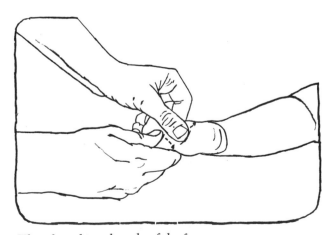

Thumbstroking the sole of the foot.

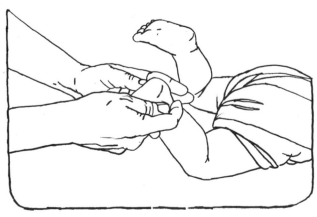

Circling the ankle bones.

Circle the ankle bones. Using your fingertips, slowly and very gently circle around both ankle bones at the same time. Do six times.

Leg warmer three times.

Thumbstroking the back of the leg. Just above the ankle, begin thumbstroking the calf muscles. When you reach the top of the calf, change your position by sitting opposite the knee. Continue thumbstroking up to the top of the thigh. Do the whole stroke once, thumbstroking from ankle to buttock, using medium to firm pressure. Go slowly, so this takes a minute. Now move back to sitting at the foot of the bed.

Optional variations:
Mentally divide the calf and thigh into three sections (inside, top and outside); thumbstroke each section separately.

   Combine raking and thumbstroking the calf, then combine raking and thumbstroking the thigh.

Leg warmer ten times.

Basic relaxation sequence.
Now move to the other leg and repeat this series of strokes.

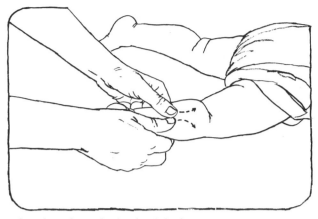

Thumbstroking the back of the leg.

Back of Leg Massage Checklist

✓ Basic relaxation sequence.
✓ Apply oil or lotion.
✓ Leg warmer ten times.
✓ Raking the back of the leg one minute.
✓ Leg warmer three times.
✓ Thumbstroking the sole of the foot one minute.
✓ Circle the ankle bones six times.
✓ Leg warmer three times.
✓ Thumbstroking the back of the leg one minute.
✓ Leg warmer ten times.
✓ Basic relaxation sequence.

Head, Neck and Shoulders

Your child should lie on his or her back with a rolled-up towel or pillow under the knees. Use this position for the rest of the full body massage. Sit at the head of the bed so you don't twist to one side while doing the strokes.

Basic relaxation sequence (see page 15).

Apply oil or lotion.

Head warmer. Use medium pressure. Begin at the center of the collarbone, with your hands palm down and fingertips pointing toward each other. Your hands will move away from each as they trace the collarbone out to the tips of the shoulders. Now slowly rotate your hands so your fingertips are underneath the shoulders. Glide up under the shoulders, under the back of the neck, under the head and off. Do ten times.

Optional variations: This stroke can be altered by changing how you trace the collarbone. You can do it lightly, or you can really grip the collarbone by putting the thumb above it and the fingertips below, using more pressure as you slide.

Diagonal neck stroke. To begin, turn your left hand palm up. Slide it under the neck to the right shoulder. Now pull this hand diagonally from the shoulder across the neck, and finish below the left ear. Switch

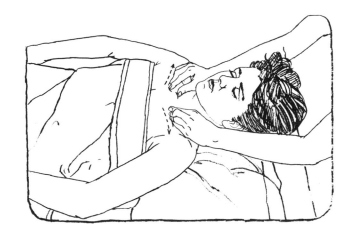

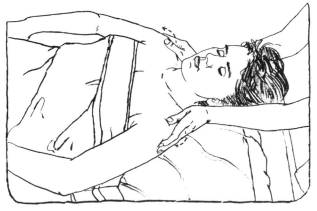

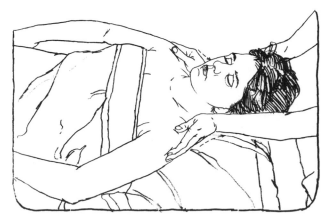

Head warmer.

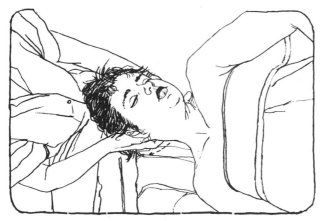

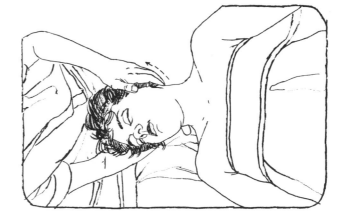

Diagonal neck stroke.

hands and repeat so your right hand will move diagonally from the left shoulder across the neck, finishing below the right ear. Imagine that you are drawing an **X** on the back of the neck with your fingertips. Curl your fingers as you slide, and use medium pressure with your fingertips. Encourage your child to let his or her head relax and be moved, rather than holding it stationary. Do ten times.

Head warmer three times.

Scalp circles. Perhaps the easiest and most relaxing stroke in this book. (Tension in the shoulders, neck, jaw and eyes will tighten the scalp.) Make a basket for the head by turning both hands palm up, little

fingers touching. With your child's head resting in your hands, begin at the base of the scalp and move your fingertips in slow, small circles. Work up the back of the head. When your hands begin to be uncomfortable in this position, flip them around so they are palms down, thumbs touching. Massage up to the forehead and cover the sides of the head. Move the scalp with your fingers; don't pull the hair. Be slow and thorough. Massage the scalp for one minute.

Optional variations: Move your fingertips very fast in large, slow circles; use firm pressure and feel for the bones underneath the skull.

Head warmer three times.

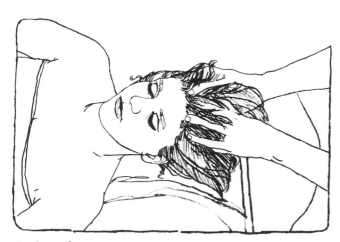

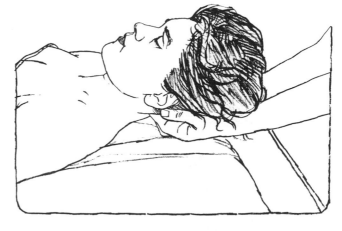

Scalp circles.

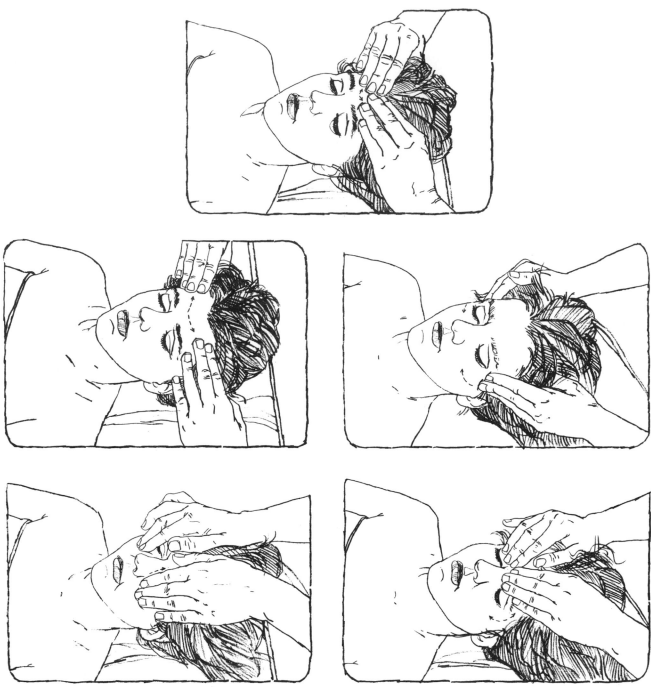

Forehead and eye circles.

Forehead and eye circles. Put both hands palm down on the forehead with fingertips pointing towards each other. (For a small child, you may have room only for your fingertips.) Slowly and gently rake from the middle of the forehead out to the temples.

Make small circles with the fingertips on both temples simultaneously; then, using the index fingers, glide smoothly under the eyes up the side of the nose, and back to the forehead. Make this one smooth flowing stroke, using light pressure. Do six times.

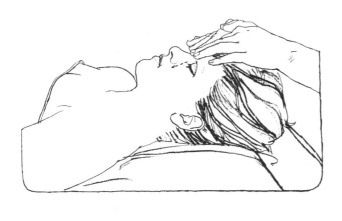
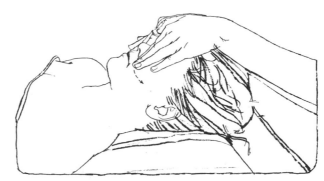
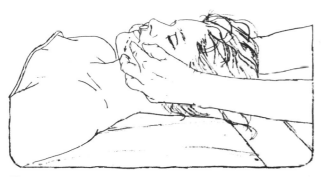
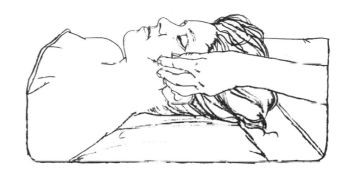

Face warmer.

Face warmer. Use light pressure. Begin with your thumbs touching under the nose, index fingers touching below the lower lip, and the last three fingers curled below the tip of the chin. Stroke from the center of the face out towards the sides. Your fingers will outline the cheekbones, lips and jawbone simultaneously. When your fingertips reach the sides of the face, rotate your hands and let your fingertips slide up in front of the ear, over the temples and up to the middle of the forehead. Your index fingers glide down the bridge of the nose to the chin, and you begin again. Practice this stroke until you can move smoothly and continuously. Do six times.

Cheek circles (not pictured). Using your fingertips, make circles on the cheeks and under the cheekbones. Be very gentle, moving slowly and thoroughly. Thirty seconds or more.

Head warmer ten times.

Basic relaxation sequence.

Head, Neck and Shoulder Massage Checklist

✓ Basic relaxation sequence.
✓ Apply oil or lotion.
✓ Head warmer ten times.
✓ Diagonal neck stroke ten times.
✓ Head warmer three times.
✓ Scalp circles one minute.
✓ Head warmer three times.
✓ Forehead and eye circles three times.
✓ Face warmer six times.
✓ Cheek circles thirty seconds
✓ Head warmer ten times.
✓ Basic relaxation sequence.

Chest and Stomach

Kneel at the head of the bed.

Basic relaxation sequence (see page 15).

Apply oil or lotion.

Front warmer. Place your hands on the chest, just below the center of the collarbone. Use gentle to firm pressure. Point your fingertips towards the feet. With hands parallel, glide down the center of the chest to the lower part of the abdomen. Now, each hand moves sideways over the hipbone, up the sides of the hips and torso, onto the upper chest and back to starting position. Do ten times.

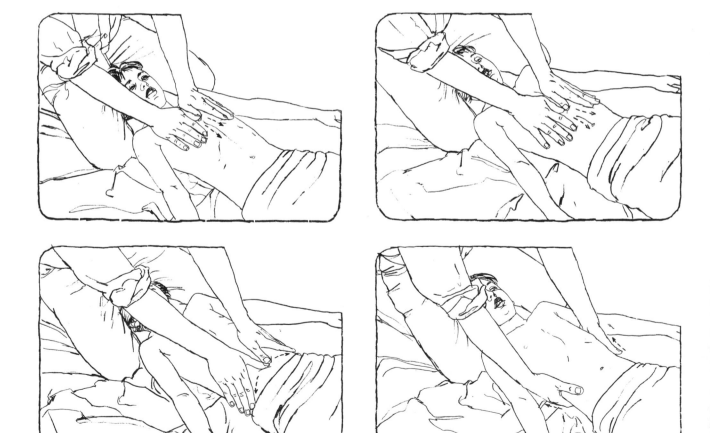

Front warmer.

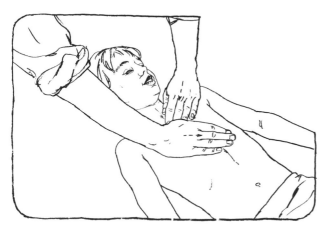

Heart warmer.

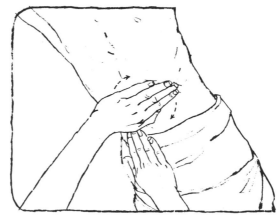

Stomach warmer.

Optional variations: Do the whole stroke backwards by going down the sides and back up the middle. Outline the hipbones with your fingertips. Combine this stroke with the last part of the head warmer stroke (page 22) so your hands move up the side of the hips and torso, over the top of the shoulder, under the shoulders, under the back of the next, under the head and off.

Heart warmer. Place your hands as in the beginning of the front warmer. With your hands, glide just a few inches. Now return your right hand to starting position while your left hand glides over the same area. Keep alternating your hands, moving briskly, and you will feel the same warmth as when you rub your hands together. The size of your child's chest will determine how far each stroke can go; try to cover the top of the chest and the area between the ribs. Keep your hands soft so they glide smoothly over the ribs; use gentle pressure. Do ten times.

Front warmer three times.

Now move from the head of the bed. Sit on the right side of the bed beside the right hipbone. Did you remember to put a rolled-up towel or pillow beneath the knees? Do it now if you forgot.

Stomach warmer. The stomach is a vulnerable area for many, so be especially gentle here. Begin by slowly making contact using the palm of your right hand (the hand closest to the stomach). With your fingertips pointing headwards, make clockwise circles covering the entire abdomen. After a few circles, let your left hand join in; it makes clockwise half-circles on the top half of the stomach, while your right hand makes the bottom half of its circle. Then take your left hand off until your right hand returns to the bottom half of its circle. Use gentle pressure. Do ten times.

Optional variations:
When the area is thoroughly relaxed and warmed, try speeding up your circles.
Move very slowly, curling your fingertips and using more pressure.

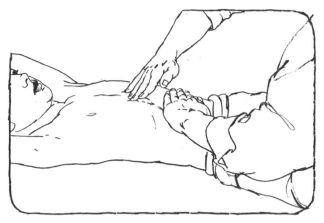 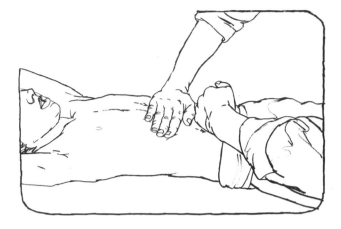

Stomach smoother.

Stomach smoother. Rest one palm on the stomach just below the ribs. Glide to the bottom of the stomach, as if you were stroking a cat or trying to flatten the entire area. Repeat with your other hand. Use gentle pressure. Continue alternating hands in a slow, even rhythm for thirty seconds or longer.

Kneading the stomach. Reach across the stomach to the side opposite you. Begin kneading at the waistline. Knead across the stomach, ending on your side of the waist-line. Do for one minute. If your child is very thin, this stroke can be a challenge—there's just not that much to grasp!

Optional variation: Knead across the stomach once, then do the stomach warmer three times, knead across again, do the stomach warmer three times, and so on.

Front warmer (reverse direction). Since you have moved to the side of the bed, you will need to do the front warmer backwards. Beginning at the belly, glide to the upper chest, go around the breasts, down the side of the torso and hips, and return to starting position. Do ten times.

Basic relaxation sequence.

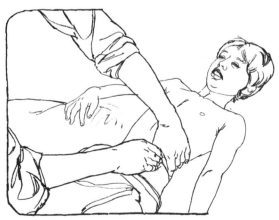 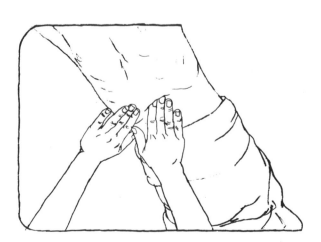

Kneading the stomach.

Chest and Stomach Massage Checklist

✓ Basic relaxation sequence.
✓ Apply oil or lotion.
✓ Front warmer ten times.
✓ Heart warmer ten times.
✓ Front warmer three times.
✓ Stomach warmer three times.
✓ Stomach smoother thirty seconds.
✓ Kneading the stomach one minute.
✓ Front warmer ten times.
✓ Basic relaxation sequence.

The Arm

Sit on the side of the bed near the hand you will be working on. Small children may lay the whole arm across your lap.

Basic relaxation sequence (see page 15).

Apply oil or lotion.

Arm warmer. This stroke is similar to the leg warmer stroke for the front and back of the legs. Begin by placing your inside hand palm-to-palm with your child's hand. Place your outside hand palm down on the top of your child's hand. With fingertips pointing towards the shoulder, glide up the arm. Keep your hands parallel. When your inside hand reaches the armpit, it will simply glide back down the inside of your arm again.

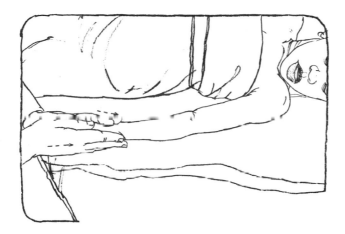

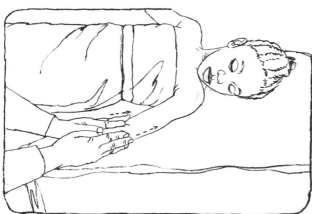

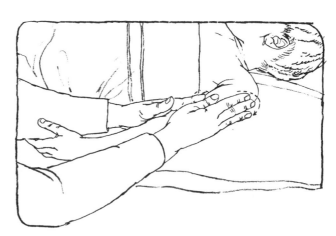

The arm warmer.

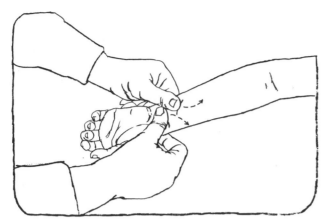

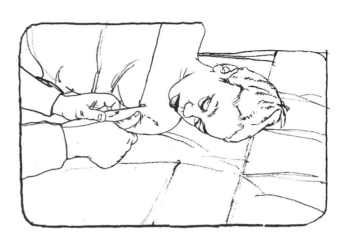

Thumbstroking the inside of the arm.

Your outside hand will glide up and around the top of the shoulder, and then back down the outside of the arm. Synchronize your hands by slowing down your inside hand as it leaves the armpit until the outside hand has circled the shoulder and come parallel to it. Then both hands glide all the way down the arm and hand, gently stroking out to the fingertips. If your child is ticklish, avoid the ticklish area. Very light stroking generally makes the tickles worse. Use medium pressure; do ten times.

Optional variations:

Use only your outside hand to glide up the inside of the arm, around the shoulder, and back down the outside of the arm.

Squeeze gently while your hands glide down, as if you were squeezing toothpaste out of a tube.

Thumbstroking the inside of the arm. Begin at the wrist and work up to the armpit, skipping over the elbow crease. Stay away from any ticklish areas. Use medium pressure. Do the whole inside of the arm once, slowly and thoroughly. This should take one minute.

Raking the outside of the arm. Start at the shoulder and work down the outside of the upper arm and the top of the forearm to the wrist. Do once, slowly and thoroughly, using medium pressure, for one minute.

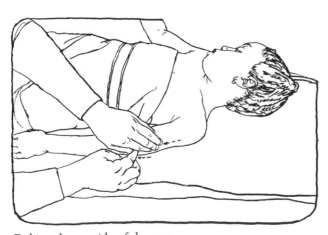

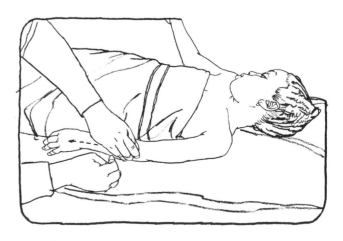

Raking the outside of the arm.

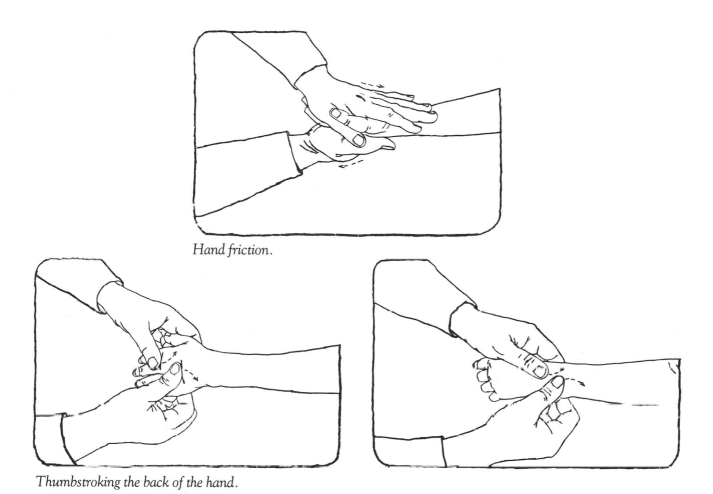

Hand friction.

Thumbstroking the back of the hand.

Optional variations:
You may make many short raking strokes or a few long ones.
Outline the elbow with your fingers, using tiny raking strokes.

Arm warmer three times.

Hand friction. Begin by rubbing your hands together as if you were warming them. Make a "hand sandwich" with your inside palm against your child's palm and your outside palm on top of the back of the hand. Now rub briskly just as you did to warm your hands. Fifteen seconds or more.

Thumbstroking the back of the hand. Beginning at the base of the fingers, thumbstroke the entire back of the hand up to the wrist. Push away from yourself with your thumbs. Imagine your thumbs are dipped in ink and you want to completely ink the back of the hand. Use medium pressure. Thirty seconds.

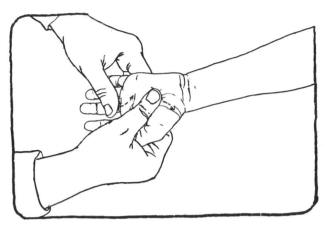

Thumbstroking the palm.

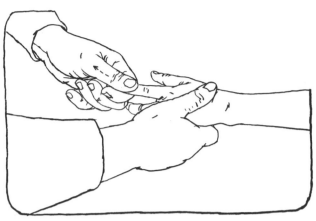

Stretching the fingers.

Thumbstroking the palm. Thumbstroke the entire palm, pushing away from yourself and smoothing out all the wrinkles. Thirty seconds.

Stretching the fingers. Use your thumb on top and index finger underneath. Beginning at the base of your child's finger, slide out to the fingertip, gently pulling at the same time. Do each finger three times.

Arm warmer ten times.

Basic relaxation sequence.

Now move to the other arm and repeat this series of strokes.

Arm Massage Checklist

✓ Basic relaxation sequence.
✓ Apply oil or lotion.
✓ Arm warmer ten times.
✓ Thumbstroking the inside of the arm one minute.
✓ Arm warmer three times.
✓ Raking the outside of the arm one minute.
✓ Arm warmer three times.
✓ Hand friction thirty seconds.
✓ Thumbstroking the back of the hand thirty seconds.
✓ Thumbstroking the palm thirty seconds.
✓ Stretching the fingers three times for each finger.
✓ Arm warmer ten times.
✓ Basic relaxation sequence.

The Front of the Leg

Sit at the foot of the bed near the foot you will work on. A small child may lay his or her whole leg across your lap.

Basic relaxation sequence (see page 15).

Apply oil or lotion.

Leg warmer. This stroke is almost exactly like the leg warmer for the back of the leg (see page 19). Use medium pressure. Place both palms on the ankle. With fingertips pointing towards the head and hands parallel, glide up to the top of the leg. Your inside hand will cover the inside of the leg and your outside hand will cover the outside portion. When you reach the top of the leg, simply glide back down, again with your hands parallel. When you reach the foot, gently stroke over the top of the foot and out to the tips of the toes. Do ten times.

Optional variation: Outline the kneecap or anklebones with your fingertips as you glide back down the leg.

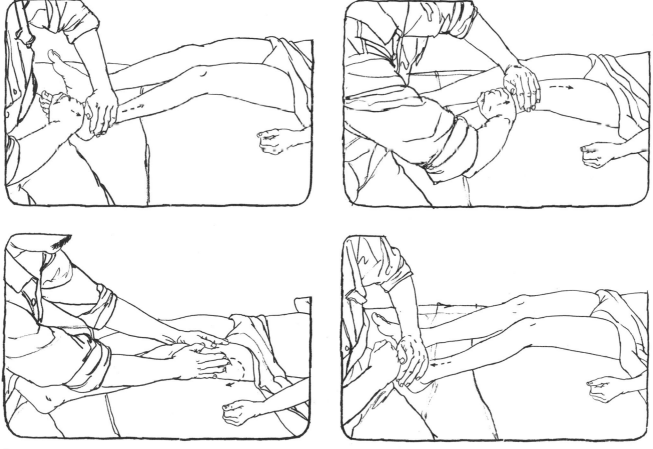

Leg warmer.

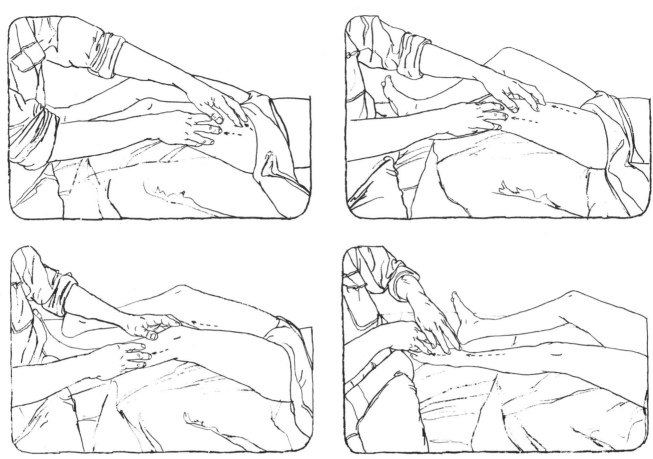

Raking the front of the leg.

Raking the front of the leg. This is very similar to raking the back of the leg (page 20). Again, use medium pressure. Begin at the top of the leg. Rake the whole thigh and around the kneecap. Continuing towards the foot, rake on the inside of the shinbone from knee to ankle, then on the outside of the shinbone from knee to ankle. Rake the muscles of the lower leg, but not the bone itself. Do the whole leg once, slowly and thoroughly. One minute.
Leg warmer three times.

Foot friction. Begin by rubbing your palms together as if you were warming them.

Make a "foot sandwich" by placing your outside hand palm down on the top of the foot, the inside hand palm up on the bottom of the foot. Now rub briskly just as you did to warm your hands. Fifteen seconds or longer.

Thumbstroking the top of the foot. Beginning at the base of the toes, thumbstroke the entire top of the foot up to the ankle, exactly like thumbstroking the back of the hand (page 31). Using medium pressure, thumbstroke for thirty seconds or longer.
Optional variation: This stroke can be varied by thumbstroking more deeply at the

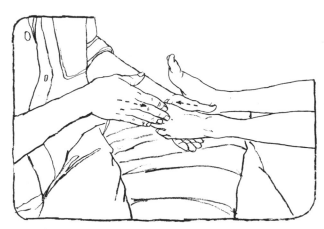

Foot friction.

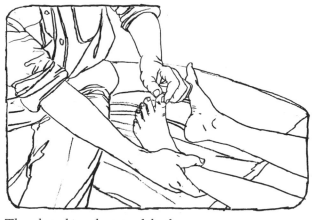

Thumbstroking the top of the foot.

base of the toes or at the top of the ankle. Imagine you are using your thumbs to massage between the bones under the skin.

Stretch and stroke the toes. Hold the foot steady by putting your outside hand palm down on top of the ankle. With your inside hand, stretch and stroke one toe at a time. Beginning with the big toe, grasp each toe and gently rotate it in a circle three times, then rotate it in the opposite direction three times. To stroke, put your index finger beneath each toe and your thumb on top; gently pull as you slide from the base to the tip and off. Stroke each toe three times. If your child is ticklish, skip this stroke and go back to foot friction instead.

Leg warmer ten times.

Basic relaxation sequence.

Now move to the other leg and repeat this series of strokes.

Front of the Leg Massage Checklist

✓ Basic relaxation sequence.
✓ Apply oil or lotion.
✓ Leg warmer ten times.
✓ Raking the front of the leg one minute.
✓ Leg warmer three times.
✓ Foot friction fifteen seconds.
✓ Thumbstroking the top of the foot thirty seconds.
✓ Stretch and stroke the toes three times for each toe.
✓ Leg warmer ten times.
✓ Basic relaxation sequence.

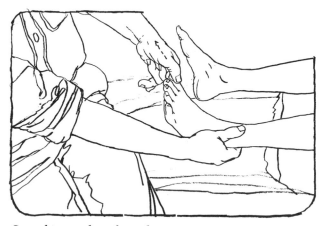

Stretching and stroking the toes.

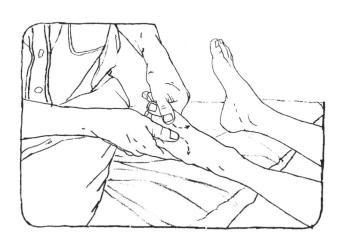

Advanced Techniques

Before attempting any advanced techniques, learn the basic full body massage thoroughly, and practice it until it is second nature. Then there are two ways you can go beyond the basic massage:

Go back to the optional variations scattered throughout the basic massage. Practice them, then add them to the basic massage. By altering your pressure, speed, rhythm sequence or hand position, you can vary strokes in many ways. These variations help you create your own massage style and adapt each massage to your individual child.

Turn to the next chapter and learn any of the massage treatments for common discomforts covered there. As you are doing the basic massage, add the treatments. For example, use low back discomfort treatment instead of basic back strokes, or use the tension stomachache treatment instead of the basic stomach strokes. These specific treatments relieve deeper tension than the basic strokes.

Conclusion

Congratulations! You have now learned how to give a basic full body massage and practice simple relaxation exercises. This chapter, the most important one in the book, has covered a great deal of information. You now have all the basic skills. You can continue to use these techniques for many years without exhausting their possibilities. With time and practice, you will become more skilled at giving a good massage. Then you can go on to integrate massage into your particular family's life. Different families will use massage in their own way, depending on the time available and their children's ages, stages of development, and needs. Massage can be a special treat, or serve as relief from stress or everyday discomfort. No particular way is "the best;" all massage that you give expresses your love for your children through your hands.

Four

Helping With Common Discomforts

In Chapter Three you learned how to give a soothing full body massage. In this chapter you will learn how to use hydrotherapy (applications of hot and cold water) and massage to treat some common physical discomforts. While these discomforts are not medical problems that need a doctor's care, they can be very bothersome to a child. Drugs such as painkillers, laxatives, decongestants, anti-inflammatories, muscle relaxants or sleeping pills are sometimes necessary and useful, but they have side effects, and tend to work against the body's natural self-healing mechanisms. Deep relaxation, massage and hydrotherapy work *with* these mechanisms. While you relieve these discomforts using only water and your own hands, you will also teach your children some important lessons about their ability to care for themselves and others. You will be teaching them that it is better to take time and work with the body rather than rely on a "quick fix" such as a drug. You will teach them confidence and self-reliance in dealing with discomfort, and respect for the body's capacity to heal itself.

How To Use the Treatments In This Chapter

You may approach this chapter in two different ways, depending on how you want to help your child, but in either case, it is essential to learn the basic techniques in Chapter Three. Then you have two options. One, if your child has a specific discomfort, go directly to that section. Once you have learned the treatment, you can do it whenever your child needs relief. Or two, each treatment may be included in the full body massage to relieve deeper layers of tension. For example, you can apply the treatment for eye fatigue in addition to the basic head massage.

Each total treatment takes twenty to thirty minutes. If you do the hydrotherapy treatment or the massage treatment alone, each will take ten to fifteen minutes. These treatments have been used successfully in many situations. If you are away from home and have no oils or linens, improvise. Find the quietest corner you can. Almost every home has hot and cold water and some kind of skin lotion you can use. You can massage the scalp, face, feet and hands without oil or lotion, and work on pressure points through clothing if necessary. Just having your child lying down and practicing the relaxation sequence can be very helpful.

Hydrotherapy: Use the hot or cold water treatment for each discomfort before you begin massaging. The effect of hydrotherapy is to increase circulation in the area being warmed or cooled and help relieve pain, thereby making the area more relaxed and receptive to massage. Whenever using hot water, be careful not to burn your hand or your child's skin with water that is too hot!

The Massage Technique: Most of the treatments in this chapter combine the Swedish/Esalen strokes you learned in Chapter Three with pressure point massage. The Swedish/Esalen massage is smooth and gliding; it sweeps over and relaxes large areas. Pressure point massage is a very different approach—individual fingers put steady pressure on very small, specific areas. It is a superb way to release deep tension, so long as great care is taken to apply the proper amount of pressure. Too little pressure will not release deep tension, while too much pressure will hurt your child, making the massage an unpleasant and stressful experience.

For each new point, place the thumb or fingers on the specified spot. Use the flat of the finger, not the tip. Slowly increase your pressure until your child says the point is just beginning to hurt. Let up just a tiny bit so the point does not hurt at all. Hold each point for about ten seconds, then slowly decrease the pressure and take your finger away. If you have difficulty locating a spot, your child can tell you where he or she is especially tight or sensitive.

Begin each massage treatment with the basic relaxation sequence (see page 15); apply oil or lotion except where indicated. End with the basic relaxation sequence.

Bruises

A bruise is a discoloration of the skin due to an injury (such as a blow) which has not broken the skin. Blood vessels beneath the skin are broken, however, and blood then escapes into the surrounding tissue. Massage can soothe a bruised area, reduce muscle tightness caused by pain, and promote good circulation to help the bruise heal. However, do not apply hydrotherapy or massage to a bruised area unless you know the cause of the bruise. Your doctor should be consulted about bruises developing without an obvious cause.

1. Hydrotherapy: Dip a washcloth or small bath towel in hot water, then wring it out. Mold over the bruised area and leave on for

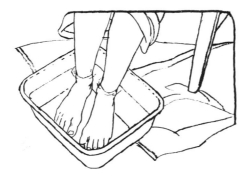

Hydrotherapy (hot or cold water).

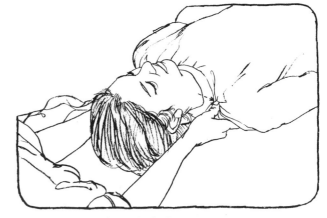

Pressure points through clothing.

three minutes. Replace with another equally hot cloth for three minutes. Alternate cloths for a total time of nine to twelve minutes.

2. Massage: Do not cause your child any pain or discomfort! Do not use oil or lotion.

Basic relaxation sequence (see page 15).

Begin stroking very gently around the bruise. Use your palms (or fingertips if the area is small), and alternate hands. Stroke upward towards the heart. After a minute or two you may increase your pressure somewhat without causing pain, as circulation improves and the area relaxes. Five to ten minutes will generally be enough.

Constipation or Gas Pain

My one-year-old woke up three times one night with gas. Each time I did the strokes recommended for colic. Each time it took less time for him to settle down and relax, and really let me massage his belly, until the third time he fell asleep while I was rubbing him. Sometimes we forget to use the skills, especially in the middle of the night![1]

1. Hydrotherapy: Place a hot water bottle on the stomach for ten minutes. This will not affect constipation itself, but will relieve some of its discomfort.

2. Massage:

Basic relaxation sequence (see page 15).

Apply oil or lotion.

Stomach warmer (see illustration, page 27). To start, gently rest your right palm on the stomach. Point your fingertips toward your child's head, and make a few clockwise circles covering the whole abdomen. Then start with your left hand; it makes clockwise half-circles on the top half of the stomach, while your right hand describes the bottom half-circle. Then take your left hand off until your right hand returns to the bottom half of its circle. Use gentle pressure. Do twenty times.

Stomach smoother (see illustration, page 28). Start with one palm on the stomach just below the ribs. Glide to the bottom of the stomach, using gentle, even pressure over the entire area. Repeat with your other hand. Continue alternating hands in a slow, steady rhythm. Do twenty times.

Stomach warmer, twenty times.

Stomach smoother, twenty times.

Stomach warmer, twenty times.

Thumbstroking the stomach. Sit at your child's right side. Begin just inside the right hipbone and thumbstroke straight up to the ribcage, across the top of the abdomen, and down the left side. Stop just above the left hipbone. Go very slowly and thoroughly, so it takes two minutes to do the entire stroke once. Use medium pressure. This stroke is extremely effective for constipation; sometimes kids (and adults) have to get up and run to the bathroom!

Basic relaxation sequence (see page 15).

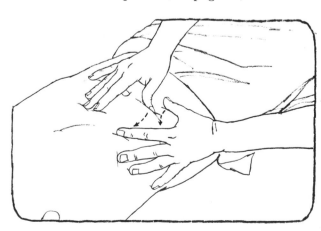

Thumbstroking the stomach for constipation.

Eye Fatigue

Signs of eye fatigue include tired, sore, dry or itchy eyes, blurred vision, headaches, or tension in the eyes, temples or forehead.

Eye fatigue can be caused by one or more factors:

• Emotional stress, resulting in constriction of the muscles which move the eyeballs, close the eyelids, furrow the brow or squint.

• Too much close work without rest for the eyes.

• Reading before the eye muscles are developmentally ready.

• Using the eyes to read or perform other near-vision tasks when there is a uncorrected vision problem such as near-sightedness, or the eyes are not working together properly.

Note that while most vision problems are treated with corrective lenses, a growing number of optometrists favor vision therapy first; this involves teaching the eyes to function better through exercises and relaxation training. See the self-help book section in Resources (page 93) for more information.[2]

When reading, your child should pause at the end of each page to look out a window, take a deep breath, and blink. This will rest and moisten the eyes. A big yawn will stimulate the eyes to water. The eyes should also be rested periodically when writing, watching TV, or using a computer. Another way to relax the eyes is to cup the hands over them, crossing the fingers over the middle of the forehead. Do not put pressure on the eyes themselves and don't push down on the eyebrows. Simply keep the eyes covered so no light gets to them. Take deep comfortable breaths and let the eyes relax. And last but not least, your child can massage his or her own face, especially around the eyes.

1. Hydrotherapy: Have your child run some cold water in a sink; leaving the eyes open, he or she can splash water directly onto them, and blink a few times. Repeat three to ten times. Or:

Have your child lie down. Fold a washcloth into a narrow strip, and dip it into very cold water (you can put ice cubes in the water to make it as cold as possible). Wring out and cover the eyes, making sure the nostrils are still exposed. Leave on for three minutes, then replace with another cold washcloth for three minutes.

2. Massage: Position yourself as for a head massage.

Basic relaxation sequence (see page 15).

Apply oil or lotion to face.

Forehead and eye circles (see illustration, page 24). Use light pressure. Put your hands on the forehead, palms down and fingertips pointing towards each other. (Working with a small child, there may only be room for your fingertips.) Rake from the middle of the forehead out to the temples. Describe small circles with the fingertips on both temples simultaneously. Glide the index fingers smoothly from below the eyes up the side of the nose, and back to the forehead. Make this one smooth flowing stroke. Do ten times.

Temple circles. Make small circles on the temples; go slowly and use as much pressure as you can without causing pain. One minute or more.

Thumbstroking between the eyes. Thumbstroke towards yourself instead of away. Place your thumbs next to each other between the eyebrows. Now stroke upwards with one thumb, then with the other. Return first thumb to start and stroke upwards; return second thumb to start and stroke upwards. Thirty seconds or more.

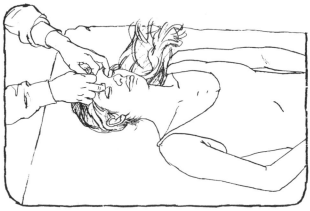
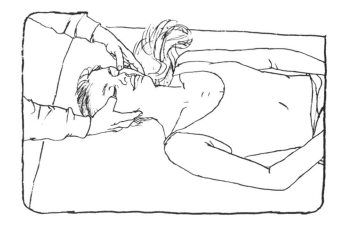

Pressure points around the eyes.

Forehead and eye circles. Do ten times.

Pressure points around the eyes. Your landmark for this stroke is the bony socket which encircles the eye. Begin at the inside corner of the eye socket, just below the beginning of the eyebrow. Do both sides at once. With your index finger, gently curl underneath the ridge of bone and press upwards. Be very careful to avoid pressing on the eye itself. Go just to the point of soreness (not pain), back off a bit, and hold for ten seconds. Do a second and a third point, evenly spaced in the middle part of the socket. Finish with a fourth point at the outside corner. Hold each point for ten seconds.

Now press on the bottom of the eye socket. Using your thumbs, do a fifth and sixth point in the middle part of the socket, and finish with a seventh point at the inside corner.

Face warmer (see illustration, page 25). Start with your thumbs touching under the nose, with index fingers touching below the lower lip and the last three fingers curled beneath the tip of the chin. Stroke from the center of the face out towards the sides, with your fingers outlining the cheekbones, lips and jawbone simultaneously. When your fingertips reach the sides of the face, rotate your hands. Slide your fingertips in front of the ear, over the temples and up to the middle of the forehead. Let your index fingers glide down the bridge of the nose to the chin, where you begin again. Use light pressure. Do six times.

Cupping the eyes. Gently cup your hands over the eyes, with fingertips pointing towards each other. Be careful not to press on the eyeball. Hold for thirty seconds, then slowly take your hands away.

Basic relaxation sequence.

Fractures

After a broken bone has healed and its cast is removed, the muscles around the break are usually quite weak. For each week of being immobilized in a cast, it takes about six weeks before the muscles regain their

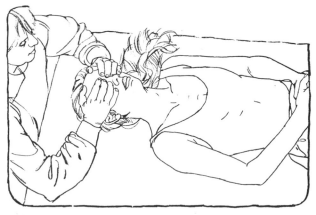

Cupping the eyes.

full strength. Massage can exercise weakened muscles without fatiguing them, and reduce muscle tightness and spasm caused by pain; this will help the child move the area again. Massage will also speed up the healing process by promoting good circulation. Massaging the area will help your child relax there, preventing chronic muscular shielding caused by trauma and pain.

1. Hydrotherapy: Dip a washcloth or small bath towel in hot water and then wring it out. Mold over the area of the break and leave on for three minutes, then replace with another equally hot cloth for three minutes. Alternate cloths for a total time of nine to twelve minutes.

2. Massage: This may be done one to three times every day. Do not cause your child any pain or discomfort!

Basic relaxation sequence (see page 15).

Apply oil or lotion.

Stroke very gently around the fracture site. Use your palms (or fingertips if the area is small) and alternate hands. Stroke upwards towards the heart. If the fracture site is not sensitive, you may begin to stroke gently over it. After a minute or two, you may use more pressure, as much as you can without causing discomfort. Do for five minutes total.

Thumbstroking around the fracture site. Make short vertical pushes towards the heart. Cover the fracture site and a few inches around it. Use medium pressure. Do for two minutes.

Warm above and below the fracture site. Use your palms and warm farther away from the fracture. For example, if the elbow was fractured, massage the entire upper arm, and the forearm and hand. Use medium pressure; massage for two or three minutes.

Basic relaxation sequence.

Growing Pains in the Legs

My son has growing pains in his legs, and he often asks me to rub them before he goes to sleep. Sometimes his legs are sore from playing soccer. Massage helps, even though his legs are ticklish too.—Father of a 13-year-old boy[3]

As many as one third of all children may suffer growing pains, especially during periods of rapid growth (ages 3-6 and 8-12). At the end of the day, the combination of this rapid growth and physical activity may result in pain. Aspirin or acetaminophen is often prescribed, but heat and massage are just as effective.

1. Hydrotherapy: Fill two deep buckets or washtubs with water, one hot and one cold (put in a few ice cubes). Put both feet in the hot water for three minutes. Put both feet in the cold water for one minute. Repeat hot and cold. Dry the feet.

2. Massage:

Basic relaxation sequence (see page 15).

Apply oil or lotion.

Raking the back of the leg, two minutes *(see illustration, page 20).* Place yourself next to the back of the knee. Rake from the top of the buttock to the back of the knee. Do not press on the back of the knee itself. Cover the muscles of the inner thigh, top of the thigh, and outside of the thigh. Move back to the foot of the bed. Rake from the top of the calf to the ankle. Do the whole stroke once from buttock to ankle, using medium pressure. Do it slowly, taking a full minute to rake the entire area once.

Thumbstroking the back of the leg (see illustration, page 21). Use medium-to-firm pressure. Thumbstroke the calf muscles, starting just above the ankle. When you get to the top of the calf, sit opposite the knee and continue thumbstroking upward to the top of the thigh. The whole stroke from ankle to buttock should take two minutes.

Raking the back of the leg, two minutes.

Basic relaxation sequence.

Insomnia

Mariah has only two speeds—on and off. She has always had a terribly hard time falling asleep. When we started doing massage with her at age seven, it was, really, a minor miracle!
—Mother of a 12-year-old girl[4]

1. Hydrotherapy: Have your child take a twenty-minute warm—*not hot*—bath.

2. Massage: Begin with your child lying face down.

Basic relaxation sequence (see page 15).

Apply oil or lotion.

Back warmer (see illustration, page 17). Put your hands on the lower back, palms down. With your hands parallel on either side of the spine, and your fingers pointing up toward the head. Glide along the middle of the back and between the shoulder blades to the base of the neck. Let your hands glide out to the tip of each shoulder, down the sides of the trunk to the bottom of the buttocks, and back to where they began. Make each hand move in a large oval shape. Use gentle pressure. Do twenty times. Now move to the head as your child rolls over. *Head warmer (see illustration, page 22).* Start at the center of the collarbone, palms down and fingertips pointing toward each other.

Move your hands away from each other and follow the collarbone out to the tips of the shoulders. Rotate your hands slowly so the fingertips go underneath the shoulders. Slide your hands from the shoulders, along the back of the neck, under the head and off. Use medium pressure. Do ten times.

Diagonal neck stroke (see illustration, page 23). Use medium pressure. Encourage your child to relax and let his or her head be moved, rather than holding it stationary. Start with your left hand palm up. Slide it under the neck to the right shoulder. Pull it diagonally across the neck, finishing below the left ear. Switch hands and repeat, so your right hand moves diagonally from the left shoulder across the neck and finishes below the right ear. This move describes an X on the back of the neck. Curl your fingers as you slide. Do ten times.

Head warmer, ten times.

Scalp circles (like a shampoo) *(see illustration, page 23).* Turn both hands palm up, little fingers touching, to form a basket in which your child's head rests. Start at the base of the scalp and work up the back of the head, moving your fingertips in slow, small circles. If your hands become uncomfortable, rotate them so the palms are down and the thumbs touch. Move the scalp with your fingers; be careful not to pull any hair. Massage the sides of the head and the forehead. One minute.

Pressure points around the eyes (see illustration, page 41). Be extremely careful to avoid pressing on the eye itself. The guide for this stroke is the bony socket encircling the eye. Start with your index fingers at the inside corner of the eye sockets, just below the beginning of the eyebrows. Do both sides at once. Gently curl underneath the ridge of bone and press upwards. Press until it feels sore, not painful; back off a little and hold for ten seconds, using your middle finger. Do a second and a third point, evenly spaced in the middle part of the socket. Finish with a fourth point at the outside corner. Hold each point for ten seconds.

Basic relaxation sequence.

Leg Cramps

Leg cramps in the hamstrings, calves or foot can be very painful. When the cramp occurs you don't have time for any elaborate treatments; you want to grab the area and massage it fast! To prevent cramping, massage the area once or twice a day until it is very flexible.

1. Hydrotherapy: There isn't time for hydrotherapy while your child has the cramp, but soaking the area in a hot bath, and then stretching it, can help prevent future cramping.

2. Massage: Have your child lie face down on a bed or the floor. There's no time to use the basic relaxation sequence, or apply oil or lotion.

   In the event of a hamstring or calf cramp, briefly do warming strokes with firm pressure, then knead with firm pressure. When the cramp is gone, do a few more warming strokes, gradually lightening your pressure. For a foot cramp, thumbstroke the area of the cramp on the sole of the foot. Use firm

pressure. You may also use your knuckles. Make a loose fist and rub rapidly up and down, from heel to big toe. Use firm pressure. This will stretch the muscles on the sole of the foot. Return to thumbstroking if the cramp is not gone.

Low Back Strain and Fatigue

Discomfort in the low back area can be caused by overexertion such as heavy lifting or vigorous sports. It responds very well to hydrotherapy and massage.

1. Hydrotherapy: Dip a medium-sized towel in hot water. Wring out and place across the lower back. Cover the towel with a plastic bag (to keep the heat in) and leave the towel on the back for ten minutes. Now take the towel off and apply an ice pack for five minutes. Take the ice pack off and apply another hot towel for ten minutes.

2. Massage:

Basic relaxation sequence (see page 15).

Apply oil or lotion.

Back warmer (see illustration, page 17). Put your hands on the lower back, palms down. With your hands parallel on either side of the spine, and your fingers pointing up toward the head. Glide along the middle of the back and between the shoulder blades to the base of the neck. Let your hands glide out to the tip of each shoulder, down the sides of the trunk to the bottom of the buttocks, and back to where they began. Make each hand move in a large oval shape. Use firm pressure, especially in the low back area. Do twenty times.

Thumbstroking the lower back (see illustration, page 18). Just below the waistline, the back of the hipbone curves around and meets the sacrum, a triangular-shaped bone at the

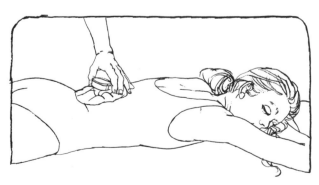

Using an icepack for lower back strain.

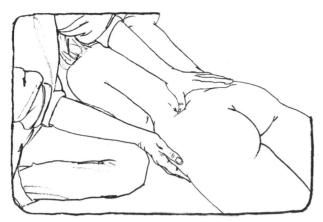

Pressure points along the back of the hipbone.

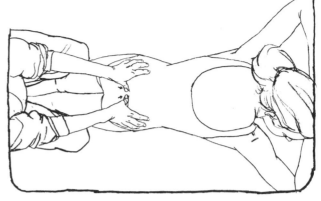

Pressure points on the sacrum.

bottom of the spine. Beginning at the sacrum, use both thumbs to outline one hipbone at a time. Use medium to firm pressure. Push away from you, first with the flat of one thumb and then with the other. Let these small pushes or strokes overlap slightly, and gradually slide out along the bone, all the way out to the side of the buttock. Imagine that you can define its shape with your thumbs. Do one whole side and repeat on the other, then use thumbstroke directly on top of the sacrum. Do once, slowly and thoroughly, taking approximately one minute.

Kneading the buttocks (see illustration, page 18). Knead the buttock muscles from the sacrum out to the side of the hip. Do one buttock, then the other. Use medium pressure. Do each buttock for thirty seconds or more.

Pressure points along the back of the hipbone. Press against the back of the hipbone, beginning just to the side of the spine. Use your thumb and press downward (toward the feet). This will contact the large back muscles which attach on the back of the hipbone. Do four points along the hipbone, each one farther away from the spine.

Pressure points on the sacrum. Sit next to your child opposite his or her lower back, or

kneel and straddle his or her thighs. Beginning at the tailbone, press with the flat of your thumbs along the side of the vertebrae. Begin with slight pressure and gradually increase to the point of soreness (not pain). Back off a bit, then hold for ten seconds. Go from the tailbone to the waist, moving upward about a thumb print at a time.

Back warmer, ten times.

Menstrual Cramps

If you are not at home and do not have the time or materials for hydrotherapy and massage, you may do just the pressure points. Teach your daughter to do them on herself as well. Do the hydrotherapy and massage before the menses begin, and the cramps may be lessened.

1. Hydrotherapy: Take a ten- to twenty-minute hot bath with feet out of the water. Or:

Dip a medium-size towel in hot water. Wring out and place across the lower abdomen. Do not burn your hand or your daughter's skin with water that is too hot! Leave towel on three minutes. Dip another medium-size towel in cold water; use ice to make it as cold as possible. Wring it out and place across the lower abdomen. Leave the towel on one minute. Repeat the applica-

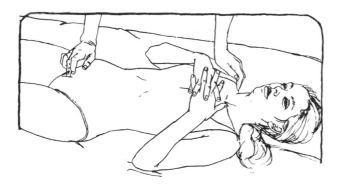

Pressure points on the pubic bone.

tion of hot and cold towels, and finish with one more hot towel for three minutes.

2. Massage: Sit on the right side of the bed opposite the hipbone.

Basic relaxation sequence (see page 15).

Apply oil or lotion.

Stomach warmer (see illustration, page 27). Use gentle pressure. First, slowly make contact using the palm of your right hand, the hand closest to the stomach. With your fingertips pointing headwards, make clockwise circles covering the whole abdomen. After a few circles, let your left hand start making clockwise half-circles on the top half of the stomach, while your right hand makes the bottom half of its circle. Lift your left hand off until your right hand returns to the bottom half of its circle. Do ten times.

Stomach smoother (see illustration, page 28). Rest one palm on the stomach just below the ribs; glide the hand gently and slowly to the bottom of the stomach. Repeat with your other hand; alternate hands in a slow, even rhythm. Do twenty times.

Pressure points on the pubic bone. Begin at the center of the pubic bone. Using the middle finger of your right hand, press directly on top of the bone. Go just to the point of soreness (not pain), back off a bit, and hold for ten seconds. Then move outward approximately half an inch until you find a sensitive spot, and hold for ten seconds. Be gentle; these points can be extremely sensitive during the menses. Move outward another half inch and hold, then once more, for a total of four points. Cross over to the left side, beside the left hipbone, and repeat, using the middle finger of your left hand.

Pressure points on the sacrum (see illustration, page 45). If your daughter still has cramps, she now needs to lie face down on a rug or towel on the floor. Let her arms relax at her sides. Sit next to her opposite her lower back, or kneel and straddle her thighs. Beginning at the tailbone, press with the flat of your thumbs along the side of the vertebrae. Begin with slight pressure and gradually increase to the point of soreness (not pain). Back off a bit, then hold for ten seconds. Go from the tailbone to the waist, moving upward about a thumb print at a time.

Basic relaxation sequence.

Neck and Shoulder Tension

1. Hydrotherapy: Make a loose ice pack by placing one tray's worth of ice cubes in a small towel; tuck the sides of the towel in over the ice cubes, then fold it to approximately five by ten inches. Have your child lie down, and place the ice pack under the back of the neck for ten minutes. Put a plastic sheet or even a plastic garbage bag under the ice pack. Make sure your child is warm, so the ice pack does not cause chilling.

2. Massage:

Basic relaxation sequence (see page 15).

Apply oil or lotion.

Head warmer (see illustration, page 22). Use medium pressure. Place your hands at the center of the collarbone, with fingertips pointing toward each other and palms down. Move your hands apart and trace the collarbone out to the tips of the shoulders. Now slowly rotate the hands so the fingers are underneath the shoulders. Let the fingers glide up under the shoulders, under the back of the neck, under the head and off. Do ten times.

Diagonal neck stroke (see illustration, page 23). Begin with your left hand palm up under the neck to the right shoulder. Move the hand diagonally from the shoulder and across the neck, to just below the left ear. Repeat the stroke with the right hand starting under the left shoulder and ending below the right ear. These strokes make an X on the back of the neck. Curl your fingers as you slide, and use medium pressure. Encourage your child to let his or her head relax and be moved. Do ten times.
Head warmer, three times.

Scalp circles (see illustration, page 23). Make a basket in which your child's head rests by turning both hands palm up, little fingers touching. Begin at the base of the scalp and move your fingertips in slow, small circles, working up the back of the head. If your hands begin to be uncomfortable in this position, flip them around so the palms are down and the thumbs touch. Massage up to the forehead and the sides of the head. Move the scalp with your fingers—don't pull the hair. Massage the scalp for one minute. Work slowly and thoroughly.
Head warmer, three times.

Kneading the shoulders (see illustration, page 18). Use medium pressure. Knead the shoulder muscles along the top, between the base of the neck and the tip of the shoulder. Do each shoulder for one minute.

Back warmer (see illustration, page 17). Use gentle pressure. First, place your hands palm down on the lower back, on either side of the spine, fingers pointing toward the head. Slide your hands upward; move up the middle of the back, between the shoulder blades and up to the base of the neck. Now your hands move out to the tip of each shoulder, down the sides to the bottom of the buttocks, and finish at starting position. Each hand describes a large oval shape. Do twenty times.

Basic relaxation sequence.

Scar Tissue

Most of the mechanisms which heal wounds, such as an increased number of cells which form scar tissue and higher levels of enzymes necessary for healing, are in place seven to ten days after an injury or surgical incision. Collagen (fibrous tissue) fibers are formed one to six weeks after the injury; they orient themselves around the injury and grow together, forming a thick firm scar. Over a period of about one year, enzymes will digest extra collagen, and scars will soften and fade somewhat. At that time the scar is probably as soft as it will become by itself. The reasons to use massage include:
• Fibrous tissue can form adhesions from the skin to many layers of tissue below, preventing free movement of the area. Massage can pull loose some of these restricting fibers.
• Scars can feel uncomfortable, tight and restricting. During growth spurts the surrounding tissue is expanding and the scar is not, and this may cause pain.
• Circulation may be poor around the scar.

1. Hydrotherapy: Use heat before massaging

scar tissue. Apply to the area a washcloth dipped in hot water and wrung out. Leave on three minutes. Repeat twice for a total of nine minutes.

2. Massage: Massage may begin about six weeks following the injury; check first with your doctor. It may be done every day for ten to fifteen minutes. If the scar is painful after massage, do every second or third day.

Basic relaxation sequence (see page 15).

Apply oil or lotion.

Warm the scar and an area a few inches around it by stroking with your palms (or fingertips if the area is very small). Stroke in the same direction that the scar tissue runs, and at right angles to it. Do this for two minutes.

Thumbstroke directly over the scar tissue, using as much pressure as your child can tolerate. Stroke in the same direction that the scar tissue runs, and at right angles to it. Try to stretch the tissue between your thumbs. Do for two minutes.

Use warming strokes over and around the scar tissue. Do for two minutes.

Repeat thumbstroking directly over the scar tissue for two minutes.
Stroke the area very, very lightly with your fingertips.

Basic relaxation sequence.

Sinus Congestion

1. Hydrotherapy: Fold a small towel lengthwise. Dip in hot water (not so hot as to burn you or your child). Place across the nose, leaving the nostrils exposed. Fold down the ends 90 degrees from the central point so they lie alongside the nose. Leave towel on for three minutes. Now dip another small towel in cold water. (You may use ice cubes to make it colder.) Wring it out and place in the same area, folded in the same way. Leave towel on for half a minute. Repeat the application of hot and cold towels two more times.

2. Massage: Position yourself as for a head massage.

Basic relaxation sequence (see page 15).

Apply oil or lotion (only a small amount).

Forehead and eye circles (see illustration, page 24). Put both hands palm down on the forehead with fingertips pointing towards each other. (For a small child you may only

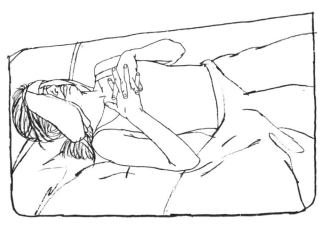

Hydrotherapy for sinus congestion.

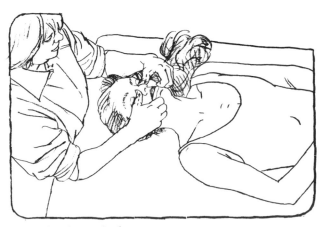

Thumbs alongside the nose.

have room for your fingertips.) Slowly and gently rake from the middle of the forehead out to the temples. Describe small circles with the fingertips on both temples simultaneously. Glide the index fingers smoothly under the eyes up the side of the nose, and back to the forehead. Make this one smooth flowing stroke. Do ten times.

Thumbs alongside the nose. Place your thumbs on either side of the nose at the level of the eyes; using firm pressure, stroke slowly down to the bottom of the nose. Do ten times.

Pressure points around the eyes (see illustration, page 41). Your landmark for this stroke is the bony socket which encircles the eye. Start at the inside corner of the eye socket, just below the beginning of the eyebrow. Do both sides at once. With your index finger, gently curl underneath the ridge of bone and press upwards. Be very careful to avoid pressing on the eye itself. Go just to the point of soreness (not pain), back off a bit, and hold for ten seconds. Do a second and a third point evenly spaced, in the middle part of the socket. Finish with a fourth point at the outside corner. Hold each point for ten seconds. Press on the bottom of the eye socket. Using your thumbs, do a fifth and sixth point in the middle part of the socket, and finish with a seventh point at the inside corner. The last point, on the inside corner of the eye, can relieve sinus congestion all by itself.

Pressure points on the side of the nose. Begin just below the bottom of the eye socket. Press on either side of the nose with your thumbs, as if you were trying to touch them together. Use gentle to moderate pressure, as much as your child can firmly tolerate. Do a second point in the middle of the nose and a third point at the bottom.

Forehead and eye circles. Do ten times.

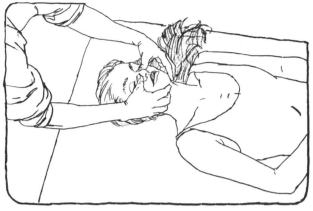

Pressure points on the side of the nose.

Basic relaxation sequence.

Sinus Headache

Many so-called "sinus headaches" disappear without ever touching the face, merely by massaging the neck and shoulders. Persistent sinus headaches then require moving to the face itself. The treatment for sinus headache combines hydrotherapy and massage treatments for both headache and sinus congestion.

1. Hydrotherapy: Use a hot and cold application to the sinus area, as in the sinus congestion treatment above. At the same time, use a loose ice pack (as described in the treatment for neck and shoulder tension, page 46) on the back of the neck for ten minutes.

2: Massage. Position yourself as for a head massage.

Basic relaxation sequence (see page 15).

Apply oil or lotion.

Diagonal neck stroke (see illustration, page 23). Use medium pressure. Encourage your child to relax and let his or her head be moved, rather than holding it stationary. To begin, turn your left hand palm up. Slide it under

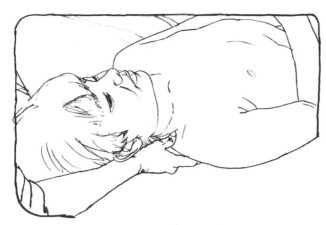

Pressure points on the shoulder muscles.

the neck to the right shoulder. Pull this hand diagonally from the shoulder across the neck, and finish below the left ear. Switch hands and repeat, so your right hand will move diagonally from the left shoulder across the neck and finish below the right ear. Your fingers will make an **X** on the back of the neck. Curl your fingers as you slide. Do twenty times.

Pressure points on the shoulder muscles. Begin right where the neck intersects the shoulder. Do both sides at once. With your thumbs, press directly down (towards the feet) just to the point of soreness (not pain), then back off slightly and hold for ten seconds. Do three more points along the top of the shoulder (as if you were following the shoulder seam on a shirt) moving away from the neck. Ask your child to help you locate points that feel tight or sore. Hold for ten seconds each.

Scalp circles (see illustration, page 23). Make a basket for the head by turning both hands palm up, little fingers touching. With your child's head resting in your hands, begin at the base of the scalp and move your fingertips in slow, small circles. Work up the back of the head. When your hands begin to be uncomfortable in this position, flip them around so they are palms down and thumbs touching. Massage up to the forehead and also cover the sides of the head. Move the

scalp with your fingers; don't pull the hair. Be slow and thorough.

Forehead and eye circles (see illustration, page 24). Start with your hands on the center of the forehead, palms down and fingertips pointing towards each other. (If you are working with a small child, you may have room only for your fingertips.) Rake out to the temples. Use fingertips to make small circles simultaneously on both temples. In a smooth, flowing stroke, move the index fingers from below the eyes up the side of the nose, and back to the forehead. Apply light pressure. Do ten times.

Thumbs alongside nose. Put your thumbs along either side of the nose level with the eyes; stroke slowly and firmly down to the bottom of the nose. Do ten times.

Pressure points around the eyes (see illustration, page 41). Use this stroke on both sides at once. Begin at the inside corner of each eye socket, just below the beginning of the eyebrow. With your index fingers, gently curl underneath the ridge of bone and press upwards. (Be sure not to press on the eye itself!) Press to the point of soreness, not pain; back off a bit and maintain that pressure for ten seconds. Do a second and a third point, evenly spaced in the middle part of each socket, and finish with a fourth point at the outside corner. Hold each point for ten seconds. Using your thumbs, press on a fifth and sixth point in the middle of the socket below the eye, and finish with a seventh point at the inside corner.

Pressure points on the side of the nose (see illustration, page 49). Begin just below the bottom of the eye socket. Press with your thumbs on either side of the nose just below the eye socket, as if you were trying to touch them together. Use gentle to moderate pressure, as firm as your child can tolerate. Press at a second point in the middle of the nose and a third point at the bottom.

Forehead and eye circles. Do ten times.

Basic relaxation sequence.

Sprains

A sprain is a wrenching or twisting of a joint past its normal range of motion. There are minute tears of one or more of the ligaments which support the joint, with leakage of blood and fluid into the tissue around it. There is always spasm of muscles near the sprained joint, and often spasms farther away. A sprained joint is nothing to fool around with! Always have it looked at by a doctor to make sure there are no broken bones. Then use massage to relieve pain and swelling, which impair healing, and relieve muscle tightness and spasm, which hamper movement. Massaging the area will help your child relax it; this will help prevent chronic muscular shielding caused by trauma and pain. During the first week after a sprain, you may massage three or more times a day, so long as you are not causing discomfort or pain.

1. Hydrotherapy: Cold (in the form of ice packs) is generally used to treat a sprain in the first 24 hours. Drs. Agatha and Calvin Thrash also recommend a hot and cold foot bath to relieve pain and swelling in the ankle.[5] (See tired feet section, page 53, for instructions.) After the first 24 hours, before you massage around a sprain, use heat in the form of a hot foot bath or hot water bottle.

2. Massage:

Basic relaxation sequence (see page 15).

Apply oil or lotion.

Begin stroking very gently above and below the sprain. Use your palms (or fingertips if the area is small), and alternate hands. Stroke upwards towards the heart. For a sprained ankle, stroke up the shins, over the knee, and up the thigh, then use your fingertips to stroke from toes to ankle. For a sprained wrist, stroke up the forearm and upper arm, then use your fingertips to stroke from fingers to wrist. Do for five minutes.

Thumbstroking the sprain. Be extremely gentle. Make short vertical pushes towards the heart. Cover the sprain and a few inches around it. Do for one to two minutes.

Stroke above and below the sprain as in the paragraph above. Do for five minutes.

Basic relaxation sequence.

Tension Headache

In younger children, the cause of head pain is frequently stress. Stress and tension can cause headaches even in five-year-olds; in older children most headaches are due to stress. Muscle spasms in the neck and scalp cause these pains, aggravated possibly by a widening of blood vessels inside the brain. Tension headaches can occur in any part of the head, produce a dull or swollen feeling inside the head, and usually come on slowly. Headaches are often the first symptom of stressful problems at school, at home, or with friends.[6]

1. Hydrotherapy: Run cold water in the sink; have your child put his or her head in the sink and let the water run over the scalp for three minutes. Towel hair dry. Or:
   Use a loose ice pack on the back of the neck for ten minutes. See instructions in the treatment for neck and shoulder tension (page 46).

2. Massage: If you are away from home, you can do this sequence on the floor, while you sit cross-legged at your child's head.

Basic relaxation sequence (see page 15).

Apply oil or lotion.

Head warmer (see illustration, page 22). Begin at the center of the collarbone, with your hands palm down and fingertips pointing toward each other. Your hands will move away from each other as they trace the collarbone out to the tips of the shoulders. Rotate your hands slowly so the fingertips go underneath the shoulders. Slide your hands from the shoulders, along the back of the neck, under the head and off. Use medium pressure. Do ten times.

Diagonal neck stroke (see illustration, page 23). To begin, turn your left hand palm up. Slide it under the neck to the right shoulder. Now pull this hand diagonally from the shoulder across the neck, and finish below the left ear. Switch hands and repeat so your right hand will move diagonally from the left shoulder across the neck, finishing below the right ear. Imagine that you are drawing an **X** on the back of the neck with your fingertips. Curl your fingers as you slide, and use medium pressure with your fingertips. Encourage your child to let his or her head relax and be moved, rather than

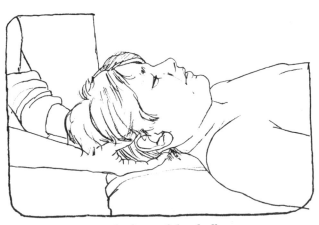

Pressure points on the base of the skull.

holding it stationary. Do ten times.

Head warmer, ten times.

Scalp circles (see illustration, page 23). Turn both hands palm up, little fingers touching, to form a basket in which your child's head rests. Start at the base of the scalp and work up the back of the head, moving your fingertips in slow, small circles. If your hands become uncomfortable, rotate them so the palms are down and the thumbs touch. Move the scalp with your fingers; be careful not to pull any hair. Massage the sides of the head and the forehead. One minute.

Pressure points on the shoulder muscles (see illustration, page 50). Do both sides at once. Start where the neck intersects the shoulders. With your thumbs, press directly down (towards the feet) until your child feels soreness, not pain. Back off slightly and hold for ten seconds. Do three more points spaced in a line along the top of each shoulder, moving away from the neck. Ask your child to help you locate other points that feel sore or tight. Hold for ten seconds each. Sometimes holding these spots alone will get rid of a tension headache.

Diagonal neck stroke, ten times.

Pressure points on the base of the skull. Let the head rest in your hands as in scalp circles. Curl your fingertips under the bony ridge at the base of the skull (close to the hairline). Begin with a pressure point just a tiny bit to either side of the midline. Do both sides at once. Press upward with your middle fingers. Go just to the point of soreness (not pain), then back off slightly and hold for ten seconds. Do two more points, moving out towards the ear. Ask your child to help you locate points that feel tight or sore. Hold the last two points for ten seconds also.

Diagonal neck stroke, ten times.

Head warmer, ten times.

Basic relaxation sequence.

Light massage with a natural bristle hairbrush can also relieve headaches. Be sure to brush the entire scalp. Repeat four or five times on both sides of the head, gradually moving higher until you have brushed the whole scalp.

Tension Stomachache

When we refer to recurrent abdominal pain, we are talking about repeated bouts of abdominal pain for which no explanation is obvious. Somewhere between 10 and 20 percent of all children will complain of these recurrent problems.... The most common cause of abdominal pain in adults and children alike is stress.[7]

1. Hydrotherapy: Place a hot water bottle on the stomach for ten minutes.

2. Massage:

Basic relaxation sequence (see page 15).

Apply oil or lotion.

Stomach warmer (see illustration, page 27). The stomach is often vulnerable, so apply only gentle pressure. First, make contact using the palm of your right hand (the hand closest to the stomach). With your fingertips pointing headwards, make a few clockwise circles that cover the whole abdomen. Then start using your left hand to make clockwise half-circles on the top half of the stomach, while your right hand describes the bottom half-circle. Take your left hand off until your right hand returns to the bottom half of its circle. Do twenty times.

Stomach smoother (see illustration, page 28).

Start with one palm on the stomach just below the ribs. Glide to the bottom of the stomach, using gentle, even pressure over the entire area. Repeat with your other hand. Continue alternating hands in a slow, steady rhythm. Do twenty times.

Stomach warmer, twenty times.

Stomach smoother, twenty times.

Stomach warmer, twenty times.

Basic relaxation sequence.

Tired Feet

Massage can bring great relief for feet that are fatigued from standing for long periods or from vigorous exercise. A 1989 study at the University of North Carolina found that a ten-minute leg massage after vigorous leg weight lifting reduced muscular fatigue even better than just sitting quietly.[8] Massage feels great, improves the circulation in the feet, and stretches tight muscles, especially in the arch.

1. Hydrotherapy: This hot and cold foot bath feels wonderful any time.

Fill two deep buckets or washtubs with water, one hot and one cold (put in a few ice cubes).

Put both feet in the hot water for three minutes.
Put both feet in the cold water for one minute.
Put both feet in the hot water for three minutes.

Put both feet in the cold water for one minute.

Dry the feet.

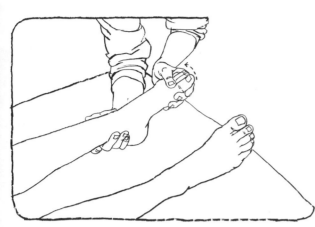

Stretching the sole of the foot.

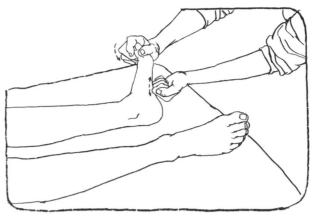

Knuckling the sole.

2. Massage: Position yourself as for massaging the front of the leg. Begin with the right foot.

Basic relaxation sequence (see page 15).

Apply oil or lotion.

Foot friction (see illustration, page 35). Rub your palms together as if to warm them. Place your left hand palm down on the top of the foot and your right hand palm up on the bottom. Rub briskly for at least fifteen seconds.

Thumbstroking top of foot (see illustration, page 35). Start from the base of the toes. Thumbstroke the entire top of the foot up to the ankle, using medium pressure. Push

away from you with your thumbs, covering the entire surface of the top of the foot. Thumbstroke for at least one minute.

Foot friction fifteen seconds or longer.

Stretching the sole of the foot. Hold underneath the heel with your right hand, and grasp the toes with your left hand. Bend them back firmly but gently. Hold for ten seconds.

Knuckling the sole. Make a loose fist with your right hand. Hold the top of the foot with your left hand. Rub rapidly up and down the sole from heel to big toe, using firm pressure. Continue for fifteen seconds.

Rotate the ankle. Hold the heel with your left hand. Using the heel of your right hand against the ball of the foot, gently rotate the foot, making a large circle. Your child must relax and not help you make circles. Do ten slow circles, reverse direction and do ten more.
Knuckling the sole, fifteen seconds.

Foot friction, fifteen seconds.

Stretch and stroke each toe (see illustration, page 35). Hold the foot steady by putting your outside hand palm down on top of the ankle. Now with your inside hand you will

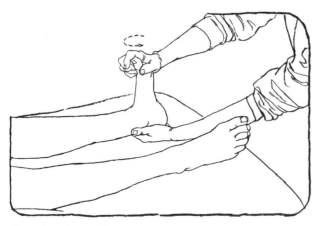

Rotating the ankle.

stretch and stroke one toe at a time. Beginning with the big toe, grasp each toe and gently rotate it in a circle three times, then rotate in the opposite direction three times. To stroke, put your index finger underneath each toe and your thumb on top; gently pull as you slide from the base to the tip and off. Stroke each toe three times.

Foot friction, fifteen seconds or longer.

Basic relaxation sequence.

Now move to the left foot and repeat, using the opposite hands.

Five

Troubleshooting

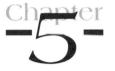

The more massage you do with your child, the easier it will be for him or her to let go of tension. However, we all respond differently to massage from day to day, depending upon our mood, tension level, need to be close to others, the kind of exercise we're getting, and other factors. When massage does not seem to be working, for whatever reason, this chapter will help you pinpoint the problem and solve it. Then your child can relax and derive the greatest benefit from the massage.

You will probably find this chapter most useful when introducing your child to massage, or when he or she is very tense. Stay relaxed yourself, fall back on lots of slow warming strokes, and look through the list of problems. Identify what seems to be the problem, then try one or more possible solutions. Often something very simple will completely solve the problem. Above all, be patient, and move at your child's pace.

My child flinches or withdraws when a specific area is touched.
1. First ask your child how the area feels.

Then ask if it's all right to massage there.
2. Gently and slowly place your palms on the area. Have child do the basic relaxation sequence, then try massage there again.
3. Continue massaging, but use very light pressure.
4. Move to an area where massage is very comfortable, such as the back, and return when your child is very relaxed.
5. Put your child's hand on the sensitive area, and cover with your hand. Glide both hands over the area a few times, then slip your child's hand out. Continue massaging.
6. Massage the same area on the opposite side of the body, giving the "flinchy" area the message that relaxation feels good.

My child is extremely tense and cannot relax.
1. Do the basic relaxation sequence a few times.
2. Massage the area child feels most comfortable with (often the back).
3. Suggest a twenty-minute warm bath, and try again afterwards.
4. Talk to your child about what is causing the tension.

5. Have your child read a book while you massage.
6. Put on soft music.

My child habitually squirms around and cannot lie still.
1. Do the basic relaxation sequence a few times.
2. Do less massage at a session—don't restrain your child. Less now often means you can do more later as tolerance for touch increases.
3. Pick a time when your child is very relaxed.
4. Some children will be energized and ready to go after a few minutes of massage!

My child is ticklish (too much tickling can also cause this).
1. Do not persist or make child try to ignore tickles. This drives tension inward.
2. Light pressure makes tickles worse; try heavy pressure with your palms or pressure points.

3. Cover the ticklish area briefly each time you do massage, and eventually tickles may go away.
4. Massage the ticklish area when your child is just about to fall asleep.

My child is nervous about being undressed.
1. Respect your child's right to privacy. Use towels to cover the rest of the body except the area you are working on.
2. Let your child remain clothed. Do head, neck and shoulders, hands, and feet.
3. Do pressure points through clothes.

My child needs a massage now but we don't have a warm room, massage oil, a comfortable surface or linens.
You still have your hands, the most important ingredient of all! See pages 37-8 for suggestions on improvising.

Six

Massage for the Child With Special Needs

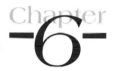

If Dana didn't get massages, he would contract and totally twist up. Some days he is just thirty-five pounds of stiffness. . . He gets so tight and hurts so much, and massage is what works to relax him.—Mother of a boy with cerebral palsy[1]

This chapter answers the question, "Can I massage my special needs child?" The answer is a most definite "Yes!" Massage not only gives comfort, closeness and relaxation, but can help meet the specific needs of children with illness or disabilities. They have high stress levels and need the mental and physical relaxation massage offers. Because they tend to be socially isolated and touched less than "normal" children, massage can be especially important in satisfying their need for caring, nurturing touch. It also supplies extra information to the brain about the position of the body in space, its muscle tension, and its movements. This extra information helps develop a healthy body image. Children receiving uncomfortable or painful medical remedies will appreciate something that simply feels so good.

The incidence of disabilities is on the rise in the U.S., ironically because of advances in medicine, which now saves the lives of many children who used to die in infancy. This incidence is also on the rise in other countries as well, especially in the Third World. There, however, the increase is caused by widespread poverty, overuse and misuse of medicines and medical treatments, poisons in food, water, air or workplace, and warfare (more civilians than combatants are disabled in modern wars).

Some general principles first:

Check with your child's managing physician and physical therapist before doing massage. Physical and occupational therapists can give you valuable advice in many areas, such as how to position your child during massage, areas to avoid (such as around shunts, or where there is the possibility of brittle bones or pressure sores), whether it's safe to work on an old scar and so on. If you are already doing prescribed exercises such as range of motion, they may be incorporated into the massage time. Range of motion is often substantially increased after massage.

Observe your child to find out what he or she likes the best.

Never force massage on your child! Begin with a little massage, use relaxation techniques whenever possible, and give lots of positive reinforcement. It may take some time, but gradually your child will learn to tolerate and appreciate massage. Frequent short sessions may be better than a few long ones. The effectiveness of any kind of massage will be diminished if the child is heavily medicated.

The basic massage techniques covered in Chapter Three work very well with special needs children; however, be careful not to cause pain by using heavy pressure or too vigorous range of motion exercises. Be especially gentle over sensitive places, such as bony areas or where there has been surgery, pain or trauma.

Parents of special needs children are themselves under a lot of stress, with a great many demands made on them. Learn to use the relaxation techniques yourself, and if possible get some competent professional massage. Others who participate in your child's care, including siblings, could also learn massage techniques.

If your child's condition is not discussed in this chapter, I encourage you to try massage anyway. I have heard of massage benefiting a number of other special needs, but did not have enough information to include them.

Another method of physical improvement which has been highly beneficial for many of the disabilities in this chapter is "Awareness Through Movement," developed by Dr. Moshe Feldenkrais. It consists of physical exercises which tap the power of the brain and nervous system to facilitate the learning of new and more efficient movement patterns and actions. This improves ease of movement, co-ordination,

flexibility, and posture. For more information, see Resources (page 105).

AIDS

Massage can be helpful for children with AIDS in many ways. It can help relieve insomnia, relieve muscle aches and cramps, and maintain good circulation throughout the body.[2] Due to fear of contracting the disease, many children with AIDS may not have their needs for touch met, and sensitive, gentle massage can go a long way towards meeting this need. Massage may stimulate digestion and appetite and help make breathing easier.[3] Most important of all, massage will help children with AIDS release tension and stress. This may be release of general body tension and/or shielding of specific body areas traumatized by invasive medical procedures or painful physical conditions.

Use the basic massage techniques in Chapters Three and Four, with these specific cautions:

Do not massage tumors, undiagnosed lumps, or skin that has open sores. Stay at least two inches away from any skin rashes, unless the child is clothed; then you may use gentle stroking, pressure points, or range of motion exercises. Some therapists recommend staying away from the armpit and groin areas where there are large concentrations of lymph nodes; consult your doctor about this.

Wash your hands before and after doing massage. Gloves should always be worn if your child's skin or the skin on your hands is not smooth and intact. Consult with your child's doctor about whether or not gloves should be worn at all times.

Be especially sensitive to what your child needs, and ask often for feedback. Gentle stroking may be more appropriate than vigorous massage. Simply laying your hands on a tight area and letting the heat of your hands warm it can be very effective. If your child is very sick, massage only the hands and feet, and gently stroke the forehead. Gently percussing the shoulderblades (see illustration, page 62) may help a child cough up mucus and relax the chest. Gentle but thorough massage of the abdomen, including thumbstroking the stomach (page 39), may help stimulate the appetite.

The basic relaxation sequence cannot be used too often; remind your child again and again to relax.

Many of the suggestions in this section are drawn from the work of Kathleen Weber, pediatric nurse, massage therapist, and project coordinator for pediatric AIDS clinical trials at Children's Memorial Hospital in Chicago. She can be reached at 1132 Maple, Evanston, IL 60202, (312) 871-6845.

For information on Vitamin C supplementation to treat pressure sores, see the sidebar on page 74.

Numerous animal studies show that gentle, loving touch, particularly in the early years, can stimulate the immune system. Though all the details have not been worked out, many researchers believe the same is true for humans. For more information, see *Touching: The Human Significance of the Skin* (Resources, page 96).

Amputations

It is imperative, when massaging a person with an amputation or any other deformed condition, to approach them with pure love, respect, and willingness... approach this body with confidence. It's a survivor![4]

Pamela Yeaton is a nurse and massage therapist who has worked in health care and health education in a number of Third World countries, including three years with the Peace Corps in Bangkok, Thailand. There she worked with the Foundation for the Welfare of the Crippled; she trained physical therapy aides, supervised the therapy of over 200 children crippled by polio, cerebral palsy and accidents, and

treated them herself. Massage was an important part of therapy. Children with amputations came to the Foundation about six months after surgery. They were taught to massage and stimulate their stumps themselves, and to do range of motion exercises on each other. Ms. Yeaton says that she saw children as young as five years old able to do this.

Massage can benefit a child with an amputation in a number of ways. It can make the child more accepting of the stump, soften stump adhesions, and decrease edema (excess fluid) in and around the stump. When other muscles compensate for the missing part of the body, they can become overly tense or sore. For example, with one leg amputated above the knee, there will be compensations and discomfort at the hip directly above the knee, the entire other leg, and/or in the back. Massage can help relieve discomfort and tension in the compensating muscles, and prevent contractures from developing in them.

Ms. Yeaton suggests ten minutes in the morning before putting on a prosthesis, and ten minutes at night. While using the basic massage techniques in Chapter Three, always tailor pressure to your child's tolerance and cause no pain. Use warming strokes moving up the limb towards the heart. Go slowly and smoothly. Friction (see foot friction stroke, page 34) is very helpful. Also simply explore the stump with your fingers.

On painful stumps, any touching may be difficult. Start with gentle but firm pressure on and around the stump; hold this pressure to the count of ten. Once your child can tolerate it, you can slowly work into gentle massage techniques. If pain continues to be a problem, consult your physical therapist, physician or prosthetist.

Do not use oil or lotion on the stump. A little cocoa butter or vitamin E oil on the incision, if it is newly healed, will help prevent cracking and drying of the scar tissue, and relieve itching.

Begin by having your child visualize the missing limb, and breathe into it while exhaling. For example, if a hand has been amputated, he or she visualize it while inhaling, and on the exhale, breathe all the way to the fingertips.

Massage the area (especially the joint) above the stump. This is a good time to do range of motion exercises on it. Also move the opposite limb.

If there are muscle spasms in the back, explore first with your fingers to locate the spasmed area. Massage both sides of the back with warming strokes that are long and smooth. Then go back and do more warming strokes on the spasmed side. Use friction (see foot friction, page 34) over the spasm but do not cause pain.

Asthma

The main purpose of relaxation therapy in asthma is based on the theory that emotional stress can act as either a precipitator and/or exacerbator in acute and chronic asthma. Relaxation can be seen as the antithesis to stress and may interrupt the continuing cycle between physical and emotional symptoms.[5]

Relaxation training is valuable for asthmatic children for two reasons. First, the stress of asthma attacks often causes a great deal of tension in respiratory muscles, and relaxation can relieve this. Second, relax-

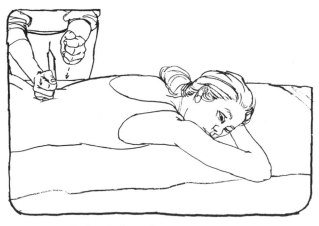

Percussing the back for asthma.

ation training may help shorten an asthma attack or reduce its severity. A 1975 study of asthmatic children who learned biofeedback-assisted muscle relaxation found they had significantly fewer asthma attacks and less need for medication. And a study done in Germany in 1948 used a combination of breathing exercises, relaxation training and relaxation massage to treat fifty asthmatic adults and children; forty-two patients showed "very good" responses to the therapy including less frequent asthma attacks, reduced need for medication, and the ability to exhale more air from the lungs.[6] The basic relaxation sequence in Chapter Three is a good place to begin teaching your child to relax. Include lots of suggestions for relaxing the chest, upper back and abdomen, such as "Feel your chest relax and get wider;" "Feel your stomach get soft and warm;" "Feel the muscles in between your shoulder blades relax;" "Let your back slowly sink into the bed."

It is also important to teach your child to breathe abdominally. Have her lie on her back, put her hands on her abdomen and concentrate on the way her hands move during inhalation and exhalation. Ask her to see how much she can increase the movement of her hands by breathing deeply into the stomach. (Breathing should still be relaxed.) You may also have your child sit up and put one hand on the abdomen and one hand on the lower back, and increase the space between the hands by breathing into the abdomen. Another way to encourage deep, relaxed breathing is for your child to imagine that as she inhales, the breath flows into the lungs and pelvis. Feel the chest and pelvis expand. Then on the exhale, let the chest and pelvis settle back to their original size. Do this ten to twenty times.

For the use of massage during an asthma attack, I have drawn many of the suggestions here from an article by Dr. Cesario Hossri, a clinical psychologist and professor at the State University of Santo, Brazil.[7] Dr. Hossri has been able to eliminate asthma attacks in most of the children with whom he worked.

Dr. Hossri uses massage during an attack to relieve muscle spasm (most common in the muscles between the ribs and those of the back, shoulders, and diaphragm), help dilate the bronchioles, and encourage respiration. Once respiratory distress is lessened and nasal breathing restored, he uses hypnosis to suggest body relaxation. He tells the child to experience relaxation and pleasant warmth throughout the body, and calming of nasal respiration.

If you wish to try massage to end an asthmatic attack, do not wait until your child is in the middle of one! Learn at least some of the basic body massage in Chapter Three, especially for the chest, stomach and back. Do it with your child, and emphasize learning to relax. When massaging the chest, stroke in between each rib with your fingertips, beginning at the breastbone and stroking around to the back. This will help relax the intercostal muscles which move the ribs. When massaging the abdomen, use the stomach warmer stroke (page 27) and let your hand trace along the bottom ribs as it circles the top half of the abdomen. Practice the massage in this section at least a few times before trying it during an asthmatic attack. Have your child's bronchodilator or other medication available in case massage does not eliminate the attack.

There are seven steps to the massage treatment, which should last no more than fifteen minutes.

First, have your child lie face down.

Massage next to the spine, from the lower back to the base of the skull. Put your hands on either side of the spine, beginning at the lower back. With the fingertips of middle and ring fingers, use gentle pressure to rub up and down ten times on the tissue next to each vertebra, ONLY ON EXHALATION.

Do more in areas that feel tight. Then vibrate or quiver your fingers on the same area briefly, ONLY ON EXHALATION. Work up the back one vertebra at a time.

Gently percuss over the spine between the shoulder blades. Percussing is done by cupping the hands and pummelling rapidly, first with one hand and then with the other. Do for thirty seconds.

Thumbstroke the muscles between the spine and shoulder blades.

Thumbstroke on both sides of the neck just next to the vertebrae.

Have your child turn over.

Gently massage the stomach using the stomach warmer stroke. Do the entire stomach, especially the top of the abdomen. Use more pressure on exhalation. Begin by slowly making contact using the palm of your right hand (the hand closest to the stomach). With your fingertips pointing headwards, make clockwise circles covering the entire abdomen. After a few circles, let your left hand join in; it makes clockwise half-circles on the top half of the stomach, while your right hand makes the bottom half of its circle. Then take your left hand off until your right hand returns to the bottom half of its circle. Use gentle pressure. Do ten times.

Massage the chest using the heart warmer stroke (page 27). Place your hands as in the beginning of the front warmer. With your hands, glide just a few inches. Now return your right hand to starting position while your left hand glides over the same area. Keep alternating your hands, moving briskly, and you will feel the same warmth as when you rub your hands together. The size of your child's chest will determine how far each stroke can go; try to cover the top of the chest and the area between the ribs. Keep your hands soft so they glide smoothly over the ribs; use gentle pressure. Do ten times.

Massage the nose. With the thumb and index finger of one hand on either side of the nose, push the skin towards the top, to the limits of its elasticity. Repeat for one to two minutes. Then very gently massage with a circular motion, just inside the nose with a Q-tip. Do not push the Q-tip high up inside the nose!

Finish by using the basic relaxation sequence, emphasizing relaxation of the feet, stomach and chest.

Autism

Massage will help relax an autistic child, accustom him to being touched, and increase body awareness. Massage can help an autistic child sleep, and reduce self-stimulatory behavior such as hand-biting or head-banging. Psychiatrist Nik Waal observes that autistic children tend to have stiff shoulders, tightly clenched jaw and mouth, and very shallow breathing.[8] She has found that massage contributes to a softer face and deeper breathing. Larry Burns-Vidlak, a massage therapist and the father of three autistic children, notes that massage also increases joint range of motion.[9] (See Resources, page 105.) A number of special education teachers who have used acupressure with autistic children have discovered that the children become more outgoing and responsive.[10]

Massage must be done at the child's tolerance. The feet and hands are generally a safe (less defended) area to begin. Showing the child how to stroke him- or herself may increase acceptance of massage. If your autistic child will not lie still during mas-

> *Other forms of touch have been used to treat autistic children. Psychiatrist Martha Welch claims dramatic improvement through intensive mother-child holding.[11] Animal touch can also help bring autistic children out of their withdrawal. A dolphin-assisted therapy program, which has patients touch and stroke dolphins, has been very helpful in opening autistic children to touch from people.[12]*

sage, try it at bedtime. Mr. Burns-Vidlak recommends combining wrestling or playing with massage. For example, while rolling around on a bed or trampoline, have the child put his or her arms around your neck while you use your hands to rub the back. Talk to your child while you massage. You may also find a warm bath a good place to massage—once the water has started to relax your child, massage him or her using soap. Experiment with pressure; for example, try light stroking for children who tend to reject touch, and deep pressure for children who are self-mutilating. Use what works well for your child. Gentle, slow massage to the wrist, elbow, shoulder, ankle, knee, and hip joints can be very calming.

Blindness or Visual Impairment

I had broken through my limitations and found in touch an eye.—Helen Keller[13]

Massage has many benefits for the blind child. It can increase body awareness, helping the child develop a distinct body image so important for balance, effective movement and ego development. It can relieve muscle tension, particularly in the areas of the eye and the upper back, which are often quite tense. It can both stimulate and relax the hands, which are the "eyes" of the blind. Dr. Meir Schneider was blind from birth until age seventeen, when he began to practice the Bates method of vision therapy.[14] As a child, he was frequently massaged by his grandmother, and remembers that the massage gave him a sense of being truly supported and a strong sense of self-esteem.

Massage can help parents develop greater rapport with their blind children, by adding a new way to communicate. Several scientific studies have shown that tactile stimulation of blind children encourages them to explore visually (in the case of partial blindness) and by touching.[15]

Apply the basic massage techniques in Chapter Three. When massaging the arms or legs you may rub one arm or leg against the other to increase spatial awareness. Encourage your child to stroke his or her body him- or herself. Spend extra time massaging the hands, upper back and chest. Before massaging around the eyes, alternate hot and cold washcloths over the eyes. See the section on eye fatigue; use hydrotherapy and follow it with massage (see page 40). Cupping is also a very good way for the child to relax the eyes (see page 41).

Blind and visually impaired children in India do hatha yoga regularly as part of their therapy program; because yoga, like massage, helps develop body awareness and release tension, these children have significantly fewer mannerisms (such as eye-poking) and much better posture.[16]

Burns

Massage can be very soothing and healing for a severely burned child. It can help improve the child's self-image, which suffers greatly from the disfiguring effect of burns. It can help parents become more comfortable with the child's body and help the child become more trusting of touch, which he or she may have learned to associate with pain. It can gradually soften scar tissue fibers which restrict muscle and fascia, helping the child feel less tight, and increasing range of motion.

Massage should not be done too soon after a burn occurs. Check with your doctor or physical/occupational therapist to find out when it is safe. However, unburned parts of the body may be done anytime to accustom your child to massage and help him or her relax. When you begin massaging the burned areas, go gently. Using cocoa butter or vitamin E oil to help keep scar tissue soft, use smooth, gentle warming strokes. Then very gently pick up the skin and roll it between your thumb and other fingers. Never cause pain! If you massage the burned area ten to twenty minutes every day, over a period of time your child's tolerance for pressure will increase. (A good time to do massage is just before applying prescribed pressure garments or just after removing them.) Then, after giving warming strokes and rolling the skin, you may use deeper pressure and, using the bones as a guide, glide over areas while pressing with your fingertips. For example, if you are massaging the forearm, glide down it with thumb and fingers stroking along the arm bones from elbow to wrist. Finish with warming strokes. If edema (excess fluid) is present, always stroke from the fingertips or toes upwards towards the heart. This allows the edema to be readily absorbed by muscle tissue, rather than lodging in areas that have little muscle tissue and thus lack circulation.

Massage can be used to rehabilitate badly burned hands. If there is hypersensitivity (pain with any moderate stimulation) the area can be massaged using progressively more pressure as the hand becomes less sensitive. If there are scar tissue bands at the web spaces or on the palm, circular fingertip massage is applied perpendicular to the scar bands, using firm pressure. If there are scar tissue bands at the web spaces or on the palm, use thumbstroking on the scar bands, using firm pressure. Also, stretch the skin to increase its surface area.

Cerebral Palsy

When acupressure stops for a week or two, I can tell the difference. It maintains a real openness and relaxation in him. It calms him down. He tends to get a little crazy at times, and he'll cry at the drop of a hat; anything can upset him. The acupressure calms him down in the evening… the acupressure is getting through, and there's an integration of physical and emotional levels.[17]

In writing this section, my sources include my own experience and that of many other

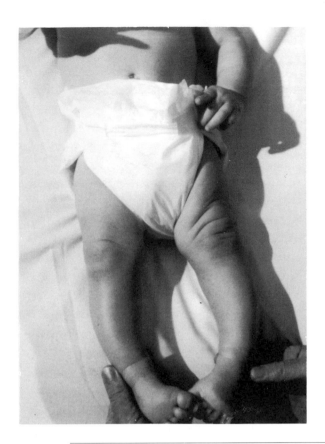 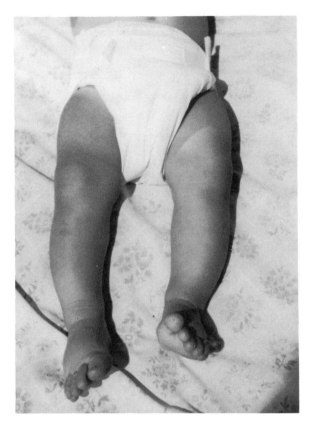

Rolfing can have significant benefits for the child with cerebral palsy. Above, the legs and feet of an 18-month-old girl, before and after ten Rolfing sessions. See Robert Toporek in Resources (page 105).

therapists who have used different types of massage with cerebral palsy children; these types of massage include deep tissue, Swedish, acupressure, myotherapy, Rolfing, and polarity therapy. I also referred to the pamphlet *Infant Massage for Developmentally Delayed Babies*, from the United Cerebral Palsy Center of Denver, Colorado.[18]

Massage has a number of benefits for the child with cerebral palsy. Whether the condition is mild or severe, regular massage can make a significant improvement in the quality of day-to-day life.

It gives perceptual feedback to help form a complete, healthy body image.

It helps increase circulation by dilating local arteries.

Massage can help alleviate constipation (see constipation treatment, page 39).

It helps normalize muscle tone, is useful in preventing contractures and helps pre-

vent already existing contracture from worsening.

Use of massage encourages deep breathing.

It helps parents be in touch with a nonverbal child.

Acupressure massage on a regular basis has helped a number of cerebral palsied children make advances in sensory-motor skills.

Strokes over the lips are a good prelude to oral stimulation and feeding therapy, especially if your child is sensitive around the mouth.

If your child has seizures, consult with your physical or occupational therapist prior to trying massage. A speech therapist can also be a good resource, and can teach you oral motor facilitation techniques if you desire. These techniques involve touch around and inside the mouth, similar to those in the cleft palate section.

Start with the basic massage techniques. Pressure point massage, such as is used for neck and shoulder tension (page 46) or insomnia (page 43), may also be effective. Good positioning is important; consult with your physical therapist about this. The legs and back are good places to begin. On any area where your child is sensitive to being touched, begin with just a stroke or two until she is more accepting of massage. Range of motion is increased after massage, so this is a good time to do prescribed range of motion exercises. (An excellent way to do shoulder range of motion, prescribed by physical therapist Deborah Bowes, is as follows: As you are moving the arm to rotate the shoulder, bring the child's hand around to touch his or her own body, first the face, then the chest and other arms and legs and back to the face.) There are varying ideas about how much massage is appropriate, but in general a whole body massage once a week and fifteen minutes daily on problem areas seem to be ideal.

For the hypotonic child: Active voluntary movement and body awareness are increased following massage. Use bouncier, more rapid strokes. Experiment with different pressures to see what is most effective. Try using the pressure point massage techniques in Chapter Four.

For the hypertonic child: Massage will help reduce tone. Use slow, even rhythmical strokes. Experiment with different pressures to see which is the most relaxing. Observe your child carefully; if there seems to be an increase in spasticity, delete the stroke which causes it. Chapter Four's pressure point massage may be useful here as well. A seven-year-old hypertonic boy I worked with complained at first about coming for massages; later he complained if he was not coming because his elbows and legs got so tight! Facial massage can be very valuable; consult with your occupational or speech therapist for a specific program.

If your child has a seizure disorder, be very observant while providing massage for signs of petit mal or eye muscle seizures that could lead to a larger seizure. Consult your physician or therapist if any seizure activity occurs during massage sessions; deep relaxation may help reduce seizures that occur then. Once the child is deeply relaxed, things which normally trigger a seizure (such as loud noises or urination) may not do so. Massage therapist Kathy Knowles worked with a child who began by consistently undergoing seizures during massage. Once he learned to relax and breathe easily while she massaged areas that were very tight, his seizures stopped during the massage session.

Cleft Palate

If your child was born with a cleft lip and/or cleft palate, massage may be helpful in a number of ways. Multiple operations or a lot of dental work may cause a great deal of tension inside the mouth or on the face, throat and neck. The kind and amount of tension will vary according to each child's individual history. Signs of tension include hypersensitivity, feelings of stiffness or tightness, and a reluctance to use the muscles in the tight area. Not only is this tension uncomfortable; it can interfere with swallowing, closing the mouth, and speaking. If your child has low sensitivity—less feeling than normal—around the mouth and nose, or inside the mouth, massage may help activate the muscles by stimulating the skin over them. (Your child may really appreciate basic massage after going to the orthodontist.) Massage around the nose and cheeks can help the sinuses drain, and can also decrease long-term swelling found near a scar.

For general relaxation, use the basic massage techniques in Chapter Three. Do the basic massage for the head, neck, and shoulders. Be firm but gentle on the face, and especially careful not to do too much.

Spend more time massaging the chest, especially the upper part of the chest just below the collarbones. When you feel that your child is able to relax and enjoy the basic massage, then begin to work more specifically on the face itself. (Be sure to check with your child's physician, physical therapist, or speech therapist first. Massage should not be done around an incision until it is completely healed).

When massaging the face, be careful not to use too much pressure or massage for too long. Do the face strokes from the head, neck, and shoulders section of Chapter Three, and add *thumbs alongside nose* and *pressure points on side of nose* from the sinus congestion treatment (page 49). Also make gentle circles around the mouth with your fingertips. Always do both sides of the face!

If you wish to work inside the mouth, make sure that your hands are clean, and explain what you are doing before you begin. A good way to introduce your child to massage in this area is to rub the outer gums briefly before or after toothbrushing. (Toothbrushing, by the way, is a form of gum massage; although its primary purpose is cleanliness and removal of plaque from the teeth, it also increases blood circulation and lymph drainage to the gums. This is why toothbrushing is sometimes prescribed for enlarged or infected gums.) Be gentle as you massage the inside of your child's mouth, and remember that even adults who understand the purpose of this are not overly fond of it!

Begin by stroking the outer gums of both the top and bottom teeth with your index or middle finger. A common area of sensitivity is the area right behind where a cleft lip was sewn together. Next stroke the inner gums of the top and bottom teeth. Now use one index or middle finger to stroke the hard palate (roof of the mouth). Begin at the back of the hard palate, but not so far back as to cause your child to gag! Stroke straight forward until you reach just

behind the front teeth. Do four to six strokes so that you have covered the width of the hard palate. At first, do a little massage rather than a lot, and your child's tolerance will gradually increase.

Cystic Fibrosis

Massage can benefit children with cystic fibrosis, especially for general relaxation (very important since many children with CF get no exercise), relief from insomnia, and soothing the back after vigorous physiotherapy. The mother of one baby with cystic fibrosis commented that massaging her daughter helped relieve coldness, abdominal pain and extreme body tension; most important, it helped her accept her child's condition and enjoy her as a person.

Begin with the basic relaxation sequence; follow by having the child visualize that as he or she inhales, the breath flows into the lungs, then down into the pelvis. Feel the chest and pelvis expand. Then on the exhalation, let the chest and pelvis settle back. Repeat ten to twenty times before beginning massage. You may massage the whole body, using the methods in Chapter Three; if not, be sure to do the back. When massaging the chest and stomach, stroke in between the ribs and along the bottom ribs as described in the section on asthma (page 62); this will increase rib mobility. Also stretch the ribcage muscles by bringing one arm at a time across the chest and gently pulling it. Conclude with the visualization of the breath flowing into the pelvis on the inhalation.

Deafness

A number of studies have found that children who are deaf can increase in language skills and/or sleep times after a massage program.[19] Massage can also benefit the deaf child by developing awareness of the body—giving more of a feeling for a body that the child cannot hear. In addition to basic massage, spend extra time on the face—particularly around the ears—and the scalp. And talk to your child as you massage.

Developmental Delay

Massage was an important aspect of the work we did. Most of the children were very tense and tight and also restless; so in order to get them to cooperate at all, we first had to get them relaxed. It was easier to begin the massage very slowly, introducing them to what we were going to do nonverbally (through our loving attitude, gentleness, facial expressions) and verbally (in calm, soothing tones and low, modulated voice).—Teacher of a yoga class at a preschool program for severely developmentally disabled children five to eight years old[20]

In preparing to write this section, I had an extensive interview with Kathy Knowles, a massage therapist who had just completed ten years of work at the Pearl Buck Center in Eugene, Oregon.[21] Pearl Buck is an education and training center for developmentally disabled adults and children, and maintained for many years an acupressure massage treatment program for children. Kathy's work was primarily with profoundly retarded teenagers. Some had additional handicaps such as cerebral palsy or autism. They tended to have poorly developed speech, motor and self-help skills, and behavior problems. Many had suffered other traumas such as deprivation or abuse. As a rule, they had not been touched, and were afraid of it.

Mrs. Knowles did one or two sessions of massage per week with each child. She generally used acupressure, with some Swedish massage similar to the techniques in Chapter Three. The children she worked with showed great improvement in four areas.

First, they showed more willingness to be touched. Some children who had shunned it began to ask for massage. This indicated increased trust of others, especially important for the children who had been de-

A 1986 study funded by the Michigan State Department of Education investigated the relationship between general level of tension and self-abusive behavior in severely mentally-impaired teenagers and young adults. In addition to being severely mentally impaired, they had other disabling conditions such as cerebral palsy, seizure disorders, and autism. Their self-abusive behavior, such as repetitive head-banging, hand biting, and body slapping, had not responded to conventional approaches; massage was tested to see if it could offer relief from their chronic excessive tension levels and thereby reduce self-abusive behavior. Each individual was given two or three 45-minute treatments per week by a massage therapist for sixteen weeks. While not uniformly successful, massage helped in many cases; benefits noted were a reduction of agitated behavior, relief from chronic insomnia, and a more relaxed appearance. For more information on this study, "The Use of Massage Therapy in the Treatment of Self-Injurious Behavior," contact Wayne County Intermediate School District, Special Projects, 9601 Vine, Allen Park, MI 48101.

prived or abused.

Second, they relaxed a great deal, which made them feel better and helped reduce inappropriate social behavior. One of the more advanced teenage girls learned to consciously relax her back to stop muscle spasms there.

Third, they gained greater body awareness, which contributed to a more definite and more positive body image.

Fourth, the teenagers became increasingly aware and present in relating to others, shown in part by less whining and greater willingness to communicate.[22]

In addition to the basic massage techniques of Chapter Three, the neck and shoulder treatment methods in Chapter

Four are very useful with developmentally disabled children. Hands and feet are a safe place to begin; the head and the stomach are often very shielded, so do not work with them until your child is accustomed to massage. If your child is self-abusive, show him or her how to gently stroke his or her own body. To teach conscious relaxation, have the child exhale all the way out. Model this by making loud sighs as you exhale during the basic relaxation sequence.

Down's Syndrome

The information on developmental delay applies to children with Down's Syndrome as well. Here are some additional points:

It is a good idea to slowly and gently stretch your child's neck, but be sure to check with your child's doctor and physical therapist on how to do it safely. Ten to 20 percent of Down's children have instability of the neck vertebrae.

Be aware of any other problems, such as heart defects or joint range of motion limitations.

Use long warming strokes with your hands to describe the child's body to him or herself—at your child's tolerance.

Spend extra time massaging the feet and ankles.

Begin massage as early as possible. Massage therapist Leonore Horden taught one couple to massage their three-month-old Down's baby; they were ecstatic to see their baby become more responsive to them after just a few days of massaging. Jeanne Hazelton, a professional massage therapist, has used massage with her son Daniel since birth to help him relax, decrease his constipation, and help him recuperate from heart surgery. In addition, the massage helps her feel closer to him and appreciate his body.

Drug Exposure

Children who suffer from prenatal cocaine or polydrug exposure are often extremely irritable and hypertonic, respond poorly to attempts to comfort them, and have difficulty receiving tactile stimulation. Gentle massage given over a period of time can help them release tension and accept rather than withdraw from touch. Various styles of massage have been successful, depending on each child's needs, with the goal of gradually increasing the amount of stimulation the child can comfortably handle. A hyperirritable and premature infant might initially tolerate only brief periods of very light stroking or simple holding; later a longer and more vigorous massage may be tolerated. Any form of meaningful interaction is a sign of success—the infant is developing the courage to explore his or her environment rather than withdraw. Over time, dramatic improvements can take place in the infant's ability to relax, trust and accept touch.[23]

The basic techniques in Chapter Three will be beneficial not only for infants but for older children. Be careful to do massage at your child's pace; you may find it preferable to do massage more frequently but for shorter periods of time. Have your child do the basic relaxation sequence as often as possible.

Erb's Palsy

Massage can be very beneficial for Erb's palsy. Do the basic arm massage technique from Chapter Three (page 29), and include strokes for the chest, upper back, and neck. Then do range of motion exercises as prescribed by your physical therapist. You will, of course, spend most of your time on the affected side, but be sure to include the other side!

Ze'ev Orzech, now in his sixties, was born with Erb's palsy in Germany. As a child he went weekly to a physical therapist, who massaged and stretched his arm, and at that time his arm was straight and he had full use of it. His family left Germany when he was eleven years old; he never received massage treatments again, and his arm became progressively more flexed up against his chest until in his forties it was permanently fixed in that position.[24]

Hyperactivity

Diagnosis and treatment of hyperactivity have become very controversial. Many parents and medical professionals are concerned that children can be misdiagnosed when they are not truly hyperactive, but instead are reacting to stress, or have other problems which cause inattentiveness, such as a hearing impairment.

Relaxation training of various types, including visualization techniques and biofeedback training, has been shown to significantly lower levels of hyperactivity. In one biofeedback study, all students showed less hyperactivity and significant improvement on tasks requiring speed and fine motor co-ordination. Some were removed entirely from Ritalin at the end of the study.[26] Acupressure massage has also helped hyperactive children relax. The book *High-Tech Touch* cites a number of hyperactive children who were treated with acupressure massage. One nine-year-old girl not only began to act in a calm, poised manner, but could also follow more complex directions and improved in fine- and gross-motor skills. Her Ritalin was withdrawn after three massage sessions. Children's temper tantrums became less

frequent and less intense. A seventeen-year-old boy with chronic behavior problems was very resistant to the massage at first, and it took several months for improvement to show; with time, he became more relaxed, better able to focus, and more interested in his environment.[27] Another young hyperactive boy received a few minutes of polarity massage treatment from his therapist whenever his behavior became hysterical; he would fall asleep for an hour or two, then awaken relaxed and able to interact normally with others.[28]

Other forms of touch have been used to treat hyperactive children. An approach developed by Jean Ayres treats children who are hyperactive and touch-phobic by gradually introducing them to touch. For example, a technique which incorporates the calming effects of deep pressure, warmth, and slow stroking is to wrap the child snugly in a blanket and roll a ball slowly and firmly down his or her back for about three minutes.[29] Another approach that has helped children gain remission of their hyperactivity is intense parent-child holding therapy.[30]

Teaching your child to manage his or her tension levels is as important as the actual physical benefit of the massage. Use it first to give your child the experience of relaxation, then spend more time teaching the relaxation exercises. To get your child to lie relatively still during the massage, you may wish to have him or her read stories, or listen to quiet music. You could wait until your child is settled into bed. Another possibility is to have your child get in a warm bath, and use soap instead of massage oil or lotion. Try the pressure point massage described in Chapter Four for neck and shoulder tension (page 46). The head, back and feet are probably the best places to begin. Don't be discouraged if your first sessions last only thirty seconds—persistence will pay off!

A growing number of children are being treated with the drug Ritalin for hyperactivity—if present trends continue, over one million U.S. children will be receiving it by the early 1990's. As many as one-fourth of them will be receiving the medication for inattentiveness associated with a learning disability.[25] Of particular concern to parents are Ritalin's side effects, including loss of appetite, insomnia and nervousness.

Juvenile Arthritis

Massage is the only way I can go far enough from the pain, get out of it long enough to really rest.—Kathleen Hanson, who suffers from severe rheumatoid arthritis[31]

Massage is primarily for pain relief, but it can also teach a visualization which will deeply relax the joints. Rheumatologist Shaheda Qaiyumi, who directs the physical therapy department at North Florida Regional Medical Center, believes massage works better than muscle relaxants taken orally, which relax muscles all over the body and cause drowsiness.[32]

Use heat prior to massage. Regular massage strokes should be done with care so as not to cause pain. After warming up and relaxing a whole body segment with warming strokes, spend most of the massage time thumbstroking above, below, and around painful joints.

Before you begin massage, get a human anatomy book and show your child a picture of the painful joints. At the same time, let him or her feel the bones that make up the joint. This will help with visualizing the joints during massage. After he or she lies down for massage, do the basic relaxation sequence. Then as you are massaging around each joint, have him or her imagine that with inhaling, the joint expands, and when he or she exhales it settles back to its

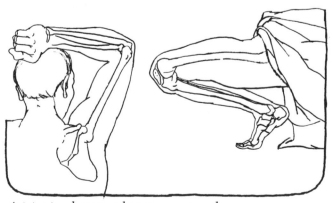

A joint is where two bones come together.

normal size. He or she should breathe comfortably and without effort. Finish the massage with a warming stroke for the whole body. Now do lots of gentle passive range of motion exercises. Your child may use the relaxation and visualization any time; the more it is practiced the more effective it is.

Muscular Dystrophy

Massage can be a wonderful therapy for children with muscular dystrophy by preventing or delaying the onset of contracture, keeping connective tissue supple, and dramatically increasing comfort. Use the basic relaxation sequence to encourage deep breathing. You may use moist heat (warm baths or warm towels) first. When using massage, be especially careful not to apply too much pressure. The tissue around joints can be tight and fibrous; spend extra time massaging around the joints, moving at right angles to the muscles rather than with their grain. When massaging the chest and stomach, stroke in between the ribs and along the bottom ribs as described in the section on asthma (page 62). It is important to massage the feet and hands. Gentle range of motion exercises can be done after massage. If constipation is a problem, see page 39.

Dr. Meir Schneider has developed a treatment for muscular dystrophy which includes a special form of massage, movement, visualization and relaxation exercises. Dr. Schneider, whose doctoral thesis is on movement therapy for muscular dystrophy, has helped a number of affected individuals to return to full functioning. For more information, see Resources section.

Polio

As a person who has had polio I seem to have two basic interrelated problems with my body on a day-to-day basis. One is balance . . . Because of differences of strength in muscle groups as well as curvature of the spine, my body and posture are rather asymmetrical. I've found the practice of Iyengar yoga to be very helpful in making me more aware of imbalances in my body and in beginning to become straighter and stronger. The second problem is stress . . . I seem to work certain muscle groups harder than necessary and other groups hardly at all. I do a great deal of clenching and "death-gripping" with my hands, neck & jaws in an attempt to compensate for and "help" the less strong parts of my body. Regular massage is very useful in relaxing and easing the overused parts of me as well as strengthening and vitalizing the weaker areas. The pleasurable aspects of massage help me feel good about myself.—Diedrich Dasenbrock, who contracted polio when he was three years old[33]

I have worked with a number of adults who had polio as children, and found massage very effective to relieve discomfort and tension caused by contracture and improper body posture. It also helps improve body image. To find out more about massaging children with polio, I interviewed Pamela Yeaton, a nurse and massage therapist who supervised the treatment of over a hundred children with polio in her work in Bangkok.

Massage can help prevent contracture if begun early; however, it should not be done in the acute stage of polio. It can prevent already existing contractures from worsening, give the child relief from muscle discomfort and tension caused by contracture and poor posture, help minimize atrophy of paralyzed muscles by increasing circulation, and help decrease bruising and pressure sores under braces. Children who sit in wheelchairs all day often have back pain, which massage can relieve.

Begin with ten minutes a day of massage for younger children, increasing to as much as thirty with teenagers. Begin with the back and affected limbs, then include unaffected limbs if you have time. (Massaging the unaffected limb gives the child a sense of what's normal.) Use only as much

pressure as the child can tolerate comfortably. In general, long smooth warming strokes are the most effective. For the back, add "back-pinching;" gently pick up the skin over each vertebra and pull it away from the spine. Hold for two to five seconds. Begin at the lower back and trace one vertebra at a time up to the top of the back.

For paralyzed limbs, start with warming strokes. Then stimulate atrophied tissue by gentle fast slapping or tapping with the fingertips. For a young child, you may make a game of this by playing "Pat a cake, pat a cake, baker's man." For a contracture, hold the part in its correct position as much as possible while you massage. Begin with warming strokes, then do thumbstroking above and below the contracture. Finally, do range of motion and stretching exercises as prescribed by your child's physical therapist. If you want to try using massage to correct a contracture, be aware that it takes a lot of time. Try using massage in conjunction with splints. However, consult with your physical therapist before you try correcting a contracture, because some are better left uncorrected.

To help prevent pressure sores under braces, rub the areas that have been under pressure each time the braces are taken off. Do not rub any area that shows early signs of pressure sores (redness, darkness, swelling, or open skin). Contact your therapist or orthotist if you see early signs of pressure sores.

For information on Vitamin C supplementation to treat pressure sores, see the sidebar on page 74.

Spina Bifida

Massage can be very beneficial to children with spina bifida. Helen Rowe, an infant massage instructor who has worked with a variety of handicapped children, found that massage could help them form a positive body image. One girl with whom she worked tended to negate the whole bottom part of her body; massage encouraged her to have a sense of wholeness. Ms. Rowe also found that massage helped prevent atrophy of important muscles by stimulating and bringing circulation to paralyzed areas.[34] Many parents are tentative or fearful about touching their child's back near the scar—massage can help them be less afraid of touching the back. This touching will also help the child release any tension held around the scar, and stretch the scar tissue. Massage can also relieve pain caused by movement that is difficult.

When using massage, be especially gentle on the lower body. It is important to massage the feet. If your child has a shunt, you may massage around it in the manner prescribed by your physical therapist or physician. To stretch the scar on the back, see the section of scar tissue in Chapter Four (page 47), again checking with your physical therapist or physician first. Caution is necessary since the spinal cord has no bony protection in the scar area, and the cord or pieces of it may adhere to the scar.

I received a letter from Marty Folin, an infant massage instructor whose grandson Jamie was born with spina bifida. He was paralyzed below the waist and incontinent; he had hydrocephalus, clubbed feet, and dislocated hips. He went through two major surgeries immediately after birth and was hospitalized for a month. His family was told he would never walk, crawl or even sit up, and probably had brain damage. He would eventually require surgery on his feet.

I had just completed infant massage training and began massaging Jamie in the intensive care nursery, and Jamie's mother massaged him too. Jamie did very well after surgery, and was a peaceful, alert and contented baby. The nurses and doctors were so impressed they began to question us about the massage techniques we were using. We've continued to massage and exercise Jamie, and it's paid off. At 18 months his body has continued to grow proportionately,

his feet will not require surgery after all as they are straightening with massage and exercise and he has no sign of the "frog leg" syndrome that usually accompanies the hip dislocation. He's very bright and talkative, sits up very well, goes from room to room without assistance, and is currently working on a parapodium brace on parallel bars. My boy is definitely going to walk! I anticipate we will be massaging Jamie's legs for years to come, especially when he's wearing walking braces, to keep the circulation good and help prevent bruising and pressure sores. As he begins to use crutches we plan to massage his upper body to relieve some of that strain. Through massage we are able to be actively involved in Jamie's healing which has been imperative to the healing of our own wounds. It has helped us keep an open mind, and gave us something to cling to when we felt most devastated and helpless.[35]

For information on Vitamin C supplementation to treat pressure sores, see the sidebar below.

The speed with which pressure sores healed was nearly doubled in one experiment, simply by supplementing the diet with Vitamin C (ascorbic acid). Adult patients were given 500 mg. of ascorbic acid (which is not considered a megadose) daily for one month; this brought their ascorbic acid levels from low normal levels to high normal levels. Patients receiving placebos instead had no such improvement in the rate of healing. The authors mention other factors that can contribute to developing pressure sores: protein and/or iron deficiency, prolonged direct pressure, incontinence, and poor local blood supply.[36] *(This last factor can be alleviated through massage—it can triple blood supply after just a few minutes, and this effect will last for hours.)*

Spinal Cord Injuries

Massage has many benefits for the spinal cord injured child, including:
- a sense of the body being more whole;
- deeper breathing;
- stimulation and increased circulation to paralyzed areas, helping to prevent atrophy;
- prevention of edema;
- less discomfort in the area of the spinal injury and the "halo brace;"
- relief of muscle fatigue and strain caused by vigorous physical therapy;
- relief of back pain caused by sitting in a wheelchair all day;
- more supple muscle and connective tissue, helping to prevent contracture;
- relief of muscle spasms in the legs;
- maintenance of joint range of motion;
- relief of constipation.

It's a good idea to apply moist heat to areas that you are about to massage; be careful not to inflict burns if the areas are numb. Massage can also be done in the tub, using soap instead of oil.

Use the basic relaxation sequence to encourage deep breathing. Then ask the child to imagine that the area you are massaging will expand on the inhale and settle back to its normal size on the exhale. The child should breathe comfortably and without effort. This can help increase sensation in areas which have very little. Larry Burns-Vidlak, a massage therapist specializing in massage for the disabled, believes that the muscles, tendons, ligaments and connective tissue need deep massage, but he cautions that massage should be done to the child's tolerance. He has massaged spinal cord injured children as young as two years old. (See Resources section for more information about Mr. Burns-Vidlak.) If there is a painful area, barely touch it at first; deeper massage will be tolerated later. A daily whole body massage is ideal, since parts of the body not directly affected by the spinal cord injury compensate for injured areas, becoming tense or uncomfortable. If there isn't time for this, some parents do ten to twenty minutes of massage in the morning and in the evening. They also rub areas that have been under pressure whenever the child is rolled over or moved. However, do not rub any areas with early signs of pressure sores, such as swelling, darkness, redness or open skin. Contact your therapist or orthotist if you see any evidence of pressure sores. Finish the massage with joint range of motion exercises as prescribed by your physical therapist.

For specific areas:

The area of spinal injury, usually cervical, may feel strained, stiff or uncomfortable, especially if the vertebrae are surgically fused. Massage the neck muscles on either side of the spine, then do range of motion for the head as prescribed by your physician or physical therapist.

If there is sensitivity or discomfort where the halo brace was in place, use gentle fingertip pressure until sensitivity is decreased.

For excessive tension of hands and forearms, use deep kneading, thumbstroking, and range of motion of all joints.

To relieve muscle spasms in the legs, use the basic leg massage described in Chapter Three, but spend more time massaging the front of the thigh and the buttocks. Use deep kneading and thumbstroking.

To relieve constipation, see page 39.

Spend extra time massaging the back if there is pain from sitting for long periods in a wheelchair. The neck and shoulders can be massaged from behind while the child is sitting in a wheelchair; roll the chair up to a table and have your child rest her head and arms on a pillow.

For information on Vitamin C supplementation to treat pressure sores, see the sidebar on page 74.

Terminal Illness

There are now a number of massage therapists in the U.S. working with hospices. After massage, dying patients almost universally report less anxiety, less feeling of isolation, more positive body image, more restful sleep, and less need for pain medication. Helen Campbell, a massage therapist in Burlingame, California who works exclusively with the terminally ill, was interviewed in preparation for the writing of this section. Ms. Campbell has worked with many dying children and taught their families to massage them. She has found that in addition to the benefits to the child listed above, massage has great gifts to give his or her family as well. Giving parents something concrete and positive to do helps ease their feelings of helplessness, and allows them to express their love in a way that goes beyond words. Doing massage can reduce the likelihood of parents becoming isolated from each other, grieving separately rather than together. She has also taught children to massage their dying siblings, and has found that they then feel included as part of the health care team, and have an opportunity to communicate their love and tenderness.

Consult with your child's doctor before beginning massage. It is almost always feasible, even if there are surgical wounds to be avoided. Helen Campbell did work with one girl whose condition, advanced a plastic anemia, precluded massage. She was held gently instead, and this was very comforting to her.

Do not force massage on the child, who is already experiencing many medical procedures about which he or she has no choice. For the first time, try saying during the evening, "A back rub might help you sleep better. Would you like to try it?" Make sure he or she is comfortably positioned, with extra pillows if needed. If the child is unable to talk, do a little massage while watching for nonverbal signs of discomfort. Use the basic techniques in Chapter Three, but be very gentle. Do not use vigorous muscle kneading. Let your strokes be long, even and slow rather than short, fast or choppy. If the child is emaciated, use only very light stroking from the head down toward the feet. The hands and feet can be massaged thoroughly but gently. Head, neck and shoulder massage may help relieve headaches. Gently stroking the forehead can release some of the tension there. If possible, help the child breathe more freely by using the basic relaxation sequence. Do not tire the child out by long sessions; even five minutes of massage can be very powerful, and will be some of the nicest five minutes of the child's day.

To a surprising degree, I've found that initiating massage opens up the way for a little humor, even with dying children. For instance, I taught a man to massage his fourteen-year-old son with cystic fibrosis; that father taught his two daughters ages nine and eleven, who then massaged the boy together. One daughter said to the patient, "Joe, which of us is going to get the biggest tip?"—Helen Campbell[37]

Another way to help a child relax is to have an audio tape of relaxation exercises on hand at all times. You may either purchase a tape (see Resources, page 104) or make one yourself using the exercises in Appendix B (page 79). When your child listens to these tapes, he or she will release tension, and may sleep and tolerate pain better. Children who have learned relaxation techniques can use them to reduce discomfort during painful or invasive medical procedures. If possible, provide a tape recorder as well so that your child can listen whenever he or she wants.

Child Social Readjustment or Stress Rating Scale

This scale measures the amount of life change experienced by a child. Each type of life change requires a certain amount of social and psychological adaptation, which is stressful. This scale is not an exact predictor of illness, because different children react differently when confronted with life change, but in general the more significant life change a child has experienced, the greater the child's suscep-tibility to illness. When children with acute or chronic physical or mental illness are studied, they are consistently shown to have had two to three times the amount of stressful events experienced by control groups of healthy children.

This scale was developed through interviews with 273 people who had many years of experience with children, such as teachers, pediatricians, and child psychiatrists.[1]

Life event scores (in life change) by age group

Life events: **P**reschool **E**lementary **J**unior High **S**enior High

	P	E	J	S
Beginning nursery school, first grade, seventh grade or high school	42	46	45	42
Change to a different school	33	46	52	56
Birth or adoption of a sibling	50	50	50	50
Sibling leaving home	39	36	33	37
Hospitalization of sibling	37	41	44	41
Death of sibling	59	68	71	68
Change of father's occupation requiring increased absence from home	36	45	42	38
Loss of job by a parent	23	38	48	46

	P	E	J	S
Death of a grandparent	30	38	35	36
Marriage of parent to stepparent	62	65	63	63
Jail sentence of parent for 30 days or less	34	44	50	53
Jail sentence of parent for 1 year or more	67	67	76	75
Addition of third adult to family (e.g., grandparent)	39	41	34	34
Change in parents' financial status	21	29	40	45
Mother beginning to work	47	44	36	26
Decrease in number of arguments between parents	21	25	29	27
Increase in number of arguments between parents	44	51	48	46
Decrease in number of arguments with parents	22	27	29	26
Increase in number of arguments with parents	39	47	46	47
Discovery of being an adopted child	33	52	70	64
Acquiring a visible deformity	52	69	83	81
Having a visible congenital deformity	39	60	70	62
Hospitalization of yourself (child)	59	62	59	58
Change in acceptance by peers	38	51	68	67
Outstanding personal achievement	23	39	45	46
Death of a close friend (child's)	38	53	65	63
Failure of a year in school		57	62	56
Suspension from school		46	54	50
Pregnancy in unwed teenage sister		36	60	64
Becoming involved with drugs or alcohol		61	70	76
Becoming a full-fledged member of a church/synagogue		25	28	31
Not making an extracurricular activity you wanted to be involved in (e.g., athletic activity or band)			49	55
Breaking up with a boyfriend or girlfriend			47	53
Beginning to date			55	51
Fathering an unwed pregnancy			76	77
Unwed pregnancy			95	92
Being accepted to a college of your choice				43
Getting married				101

Advanced Relaxation Exercises

Children and adults take in information and learn through all five of their senses, but one sensory area is generally their leading way to receive information. One student may do very poor academic work if classroom instructions are given orally, and good work if they are written on the blackboard. His main sensory area is visual, and he tends to think in pictures. Another child needs to touch the words on her worksheet or book to comprehend well; she goes blank when school work is presented on an overhead projector. Her main sensory area is kinesthetic; she tends to think in sensations. Still another child learns best through class discussion; whenever he takes a test he "talks" to himself about it under his breath. His main sensory area is auditory, and he thinks in sounds.

Because of this difference in learning styles, a relaxation exercise that works for one person may be ineffective for another. Three different short exercises (about five minutes each) are presented here, each primarily in one learning style: visual, kinesthetic, and auditory. Try all three with your children and let them tell you which is the most relaxing. The fourth exercise, Float Ride, is longer and combines all three types of thinking. Remember that the ability to relax will improve greatly with practice.

Read each exercise slowly, and in a calm voice. Your child should be lying down or sitting in a comfortable chair. As with massage, the fewer distractions there are, the easier it will be to relax. You can make an audiocassette for your child to use, or see Audio-Visual Materials in the Resources section listing relaxation tapes for children.

Waterfall of white light (visual)

Close your eyes and begin to focus your attention on your breath. Give yourself the suggestion that with each exhalation, your body becomes more and more relaxed. Now imagine that a beautiful waterfall of white light is entering the top of your head. You feel its gentle healing energy flowing throughout your brain and pouring over your face, your chin, and your neck. The waterfall of white light now continues to move into your chest and shoulders and back. It moves down your arms and hands and out through your fingertips, taking with it any stress that you have held in your body. The white light continues to flow into your abdomen and solar plexus, your pelvis and your buttocks. It continues moving down into your thighs, your knees, and your calves. Now it enters your ankles and feet and goes out through your toes, taking with it any stress or discomfort that you have stored in your body. Now you are in a continuous waterfall of white light. Every part of your being is filled with white light. Allow this energy to wash over you, and enjoy the gentle calm it brings. (*Pause one minute.*) Now slowly bring yourself back to full waking consciousness. I will count to ten. Join me counting aloud at six, and open your eyes at ten, feeling relaxed and alert. One . . . two . . . three . . . four . . . five . . . six . . . seven . . . eight . . . nine . . . ten.[1]

Tensing and relaxing (kinesthetic)

Close your eyes and sit (or lie down) very quietly. Take a couple of moments and notice how your body feels. Are you holding your breath, or do you breathe evenly? Notice if you feel any tension or stress in any part of your body. Now you're going to relax your body as you relax your breath.

Breathe in . . . and . . . out . . . and . . . in . . . and . . . out, and allow yourself to let go of any thoughts or worries. Gently continue to breathe in . . . and . . . out . . . and focus your attention on your feet. Just notice your feet, nothing else. Notice how they feel. It may be the first time that you have put all of your attention on your feet. Now, as you take a deep breath, tense or squeeze the muscles in your feet . . . hold it . . . and now release the tension in the muscles of your feet as you breathe out. And now continue breathing gently and calmly. (*Pause*)

Now focus your attention on your legs—just your legs, nothing else—and notice how they feel. Now breathe in as you squeeze the muscles in your legs . . . hold it . . . and now release the tension in your legs as you breathe out. (*Pause*)

Now focus your attention on your bottom and pelvic area. Breathe in as you squeeze the muscles in your bottom and pelvis . . . hold it . . . and release the tension in your bottom and pelvis as you breathe out. (*Pause*)

Focus your attention on your back . . . breathe as you squeeze your back . . . hold it . . . and now release the tension in your back as you breathe out. (*Pause*)

Focus your attention on your abdomen . . . just notice how it feels . . . notice whether you pull in the muscles in your abdomen. Now gently breathe in as you squeeze the muscles in your abdomen . . . hold it . . . and relax. (*Pause*)

Focus your attention on your chest . . . hold it . . . and now relax. And just continue to breathe gently and calmly. Focus your attention on your shoulders . . . Notice if you carry more tension in one shoulder than another. Now breathe in as you squeeze the muscles in your shoulders . . . hold it . . . and relax. (*Pause*)

Now focus on your arms and hands, and when you squeeze the muscles in your hands, actually make a fist with your fingers, and then very slowly open your fingers when you release the tension. Breathe in as you squeeze the muscles in your arms and hands . . . hold it . . . and relax. (*Pause*)

Now focus your attention on your jaw and facial muscles, noticing how they feel. Breathe in as you squeeze the muscles in your jaw and eyes, nose and mouth . . . hold it . . . and now relax, letting go of any tension that you may carry in your jaw and facial muscles. *(Pause)*

Now focus your attention on your forehead and your head. Breathe in as you squeeze the muscles in your forehead and the rest of your head . . . hold it . . . and relax. And now focus your attention on your breath . . . breathing gently and calmly . . . and enjoy the relaxation of your body.

(After a minute) Now bring yourself back to full waking consciousness as I count to three. Open your eyes at the count of three. One . . . two . . . three.[2]

Relaxing the body (auditory)

After I say each phrase, repeat it mentally to yourself, and feel whatever that phrase suggests to you. Continue repeating it until I say the next phrase.

I feel quiet and easily relaxed.

My body is beginning to relax more and more.

My ankles, my knees, and my hips feel heavy and relaxed.

My bottom and my pelvis feel heavy and relaxed.

My whole back feels heavy and relaxed.

My stomach feels warm and relaxed.

My chest is relaxed and my breathing is easy.

My shoulders feel heavy, relaxed, and comfortable.

My hands, and arms feel heavy, relaxed and comfortable.

My neck feels relaxed and comfortable.

My jaw feels relaxed and comfortable.

My mouth feels relaxed and comfortable.

My eyes and forehead feel quiet, relaxed, and comfortable.

My eyes are soft.

My whole head is quiet, relaxed, and comfortable.

My whole body is quiet, heavy, relaxed, and comfortable.

Float Ride

This narrative encourages deep relaxation. It can be used at bedtime or anytime a child is emotionally upset or fatigued. Parents can also make a tape cassette for children to use by themselves. It should be read in a soft, slow, and soothing voice, giving the child plenty of time to listen, absorb, and passively follow directions.

Get in a very comfortable position. Close your eyes, and try to relax your body. Think about your breathing. Breathe in . . . Breathe out . . . Breathe in through your nose, and out through your mouth . . . Now take a deep breath, and hold it . . . and let it out slowly . . .

Feel yourself sinking deeper into the (chair or the bed) . . . You're beginning to feel very comfortable and relaxed . . .

Today we're going to take a ride on a float in the Gulf. We each have a float, and it needs to be blown up . . . So first thing we do is blow it up. Take your float and blow into it, by taking three deep breaths and exhaling into your float . . . You will need to blow into your float at least ten times . . .

So now, take a very deep breath, and slowly exhale into your float . . .

Each time you breathe out, let your body become more and more relaxed . . . Each breath should let you feel really good inside . . .

Now that our floats are blown up, we'll walk down to the water . . . The sun is very bright, and it feels warm on your skin . . . The sand feels warm and cushy and soft against your feet . . . As we get closer to the water we can smell the salty air . . . We can hear the waves of the ocean . . . as they land on the beach . . . The water is closer now and the sand begins to get a little cooler . . . The sun is shining on us, and we feel good . . . Let's pause for a few moments now and feel the sun above us and the sand beneath our feet . . . Now we're at the edge of the water and we get on our floats . . . The floats feel very comfortable and secure . . . The air is warm and the water is cool . . . We are slowly floating away from the shore on our floats and we feel very relaxed . . . There are seagulls in the sky and we open our eyes to watch them fly by us . . . The water is warm and we feel it with our hands and our legs . . . The water is moving our floats away from the beach and we feel very comfortable and safe . . .

As the waves pass under us, the floats move slowly up . . . and slowly down . . . We move with the floats . . . up . . . and

down . . . very slowly . . . We feel as if we're being rocked to sleep . . . The water is pushing us up . . . and down . . . and up . . . and down . . . We feel very relaxed and comfortable . . .

As the waves are passing under us, they begin to pull us closer and closer to the beach . . . For just a few more seconds we can ride our float without having to touch the sand . . . The sun is warming our bodies, and the float ride is relaxing our bodies and our minds . . .

The floats touch the sand and we get our bodies to move again . . . So for a few seconds, bring yourself back to awareness and get off your float . . . The sand feels warm against our feet once more and we feel very good inside and outside . . . The air is warm and it dries our bodies quickly as we slowly walk away from the water . . . Now we let the air out of our floats, and the air escaping from the floats relaxes our bodies . . .

Now we've finished with our ride and our floats and we return to the room . . . As I count backward from five to one, slowly bring yourself back to being alert and relaxed . . . Five . . . Four . . . Begin to feel more alert and allow energy to flow into your body . . . Three . . . Move your arms and legs . . . Two . . . Wiggle your fingers and your toes . . . Open your eyes . . . One . . . Sit up, stretch and feel alert all over.[3]

APPENDIX C

Type A Behavior in Children

In an exercise that I once did with my third-grade class on what they didn't like in their lives, the symbol that appeared in all of their drawings was a ticking alarm clock. When I asked them to elaborate about the clock, typical responses were "I hate rushing from school to soccer practice," "I never have any time to just sit," "I don't get enough time to play with my friends because my mom has to pick me up early so she can go someplace else." In a similar exercise with older students, one commented: "I thought teachers would let up on the work during senior year, but we have more than ever. I have no time for my friends."[1]

The term Type A behavior was originally coined by cardiologists Meyer Friedman and Ray Rosenman. It is also called coronary-prone behavior, and is of concern because it can contribute to heart disease, America's number one cause of adult death.

Type A personalities walk fast, talk fast, and tend to do more than one thing at a time (such as simultaneously reading, eating, and watching TV). Their high tension level is revealed by rapid eye blinking, fast speech, knee jiggling, and finger tapping. They may be isolated from others by being aggressive, impatient, and competitive. Type B personalities, by contrast, are easygoing, can work without agitation, and can relax without guilt. Often they are more efficient than Type A's.

The importance of Type A behavior in children is that it is a pattern of reaction to stress which causes more and more—stress becomes unrelenting. This pattern can lead to serious illness as an adult. Of particular concern is the elevation in blood cholesterol levels found in Type A's, both adults and children. High cholesterol is a significant risk factor in the development of heart disease. One study found that Type A children aged ten to seventeen had high blood cholesterol readings.[2] Research at Stanford University found that intensely Type A children in fifth, seventh, and ninth grades were more prone to have sleep disturbances, headaches, sore throats, colds, flu, and allergies than other children.[3]

What causes Type A behavior? Some of

its aspects may be inherited: for example, the tendency to be hard-driving or competitive. Robert Kowalski, author of *Cholesterol and Children*, suffered a heart attack and two coronary bypass surgeries by the time he was 41. Of his eight-year-old son Ross, he says, "There's no doubt in my mind that stress was influential in my early disease onset. But the most frightening thing was to see much of my behavior pattern inherited by my son. . . Ross definitely exhibits some of those Type A traits."[4]

In addition, our culture definitely encourages Type A behavior. A life packed with activity is perceived as better than one with generous portions of time to relax. Hard-driving, energetic people are held up as role models, not those who take life more slowly. Beginning with the preschool years, most of us have been taught that the way to achieve is to try hard, harder, and harder

still. Children encounter severely competitive conditions increasingly early in life, in areas ranging from academics to recreation. Children who are are susceptible to these Type A messages may become overly competitive and stressed at an early age.

Type B behavior can also be learned, and parents are an important role model. How impatient are you when waiting in line or at a red light? How often do your kids see you doing ten things at once? What do you do to unwind when you are stressed or upset? Do you take a walk, read a book or get a massage, or do you continue going at a frenzied pace? How much time do you make for friends and family? Do you push your kids to compete and achieve in areas they have no desire to? Beware—even a massage can be done in a Type A manner, fast and frenetically!

APPENDIX D
Touch and Body Image

Body image is the individual's "mental picture" of his or her own body, its movement, and its relationship to objects in the environment. This mental picture is derived from the individual's unique physical and emotional experiences. It can be identified by the way the child interacts with the environment, and in the child's values, attitudes, and self-perceptions. Children need a definite and relatively stable body image to perceive themselves and others accurately, and to interact well with their environment. A distinct body image is also necessary for good balance, spatial orientation and precision of movement. Children with vague, indefinite or distorted body images experience low self-esteem, severe anxiety and difficulty interacting with their environment. Moderately high correlations have been obtained between a well developed body image and good self-esteem.

The body image consists of:
• Perception of the parts of one's body.
• Awareness of the body's planes: right and

left sides, front and back.
• Perception of one's body movements.
• Perception of the body in relation to the rest of the world, which can cause a person to see herself as very small or very big. Emotions can alter this perception.
• The belief that the body has boundaries, a clearly defined line between it and the rest of the world. If the individual has an indefinite or weak sense of his or her boundaries, he or she will feel incapable of protecting him- or herself. Intimacy, which involves some boundary loss, may seem to be a very frightening outside force. He or she will believe that his or her body and self lack integrator completeness. This feeling of having too little boundary may be caused in childhood by the excessive intrusion of the child's boundaries—a failure to respect the child's body as a private domain.

Schizophrenia, psychosis and severe brain damage can also cause boundary loss. If the individual has a sense of the body boundary being too strong, he or she may feel very much in control over letting feelings out; however, he or she may also feel lonely and numb. Such people are attracted to thrill-seeking behavior, alcohol and drugs to try to regain sensation.

Development of Body Image

The construction of body image begins in the first few days of life, as the infant begins looking at his or her own body, watching its movements and those of others. An infant must have adequate stimulation, especially

TT's Drawing of himself February 9, 1981

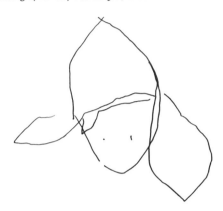

TT's Drawing of himself May 8, 1981

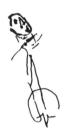

Self-portraits provide many indicators of self-esteem as well as motor control. This six-year-old boy was in a special education program; he had aphasia and gross and fine motor co-ordination problems. His second self-portrait indicates that his body awareness has increased noticeably.

Reprinted from High Tech Touch: Acupressure in the Schools *by Jeanne St. John. Novato, CA: Academic Therapy Publications, 1987. Copyright © 1987 by Academic Therapy Publications.*

that of touch and movement, or his or her body image is poor; the infant is anxious, has difficulty forming normal emotional attachments to significant others, and has impaired ego development.

During the toddler stage, body image continues to develop. Parental attitudes make an indelible impression on the child's concept of him- or herself, his or her body, and its functions. As children grow in size, shape and motor skills, their body image is continuously reshaped. During the pre-school years body image becomes clearer and more conscious. Children aged six to twelve begin to compare their bodies to those around them as they learn how to interact with others. Adolescents, in the throes of such body changes as rapid growth and hormonal ups and downs, experience increased self-consciousness and greater focus on the body.

The Role of Touch

Sensitive, caring touch can play a very important role in creating a healthy body image. Touch at all stages of life offers:
• Perceptual feedback to give realistic, well-defined body image. Persons undergoing experimental sensory deprivation—no perceptual feedback—very soon experience serious distortion of their body image such as changes in their perceived limb size or weight. The drawing on this page demonstrates the impact that massage can have on body image.
• Reinforcement of body boundaries, by increasing awareness of skin and muscles. This is undoubtedly the reason why self-touching is so common; it tells the self "the edge of me is there and intact."
• A sense of the intactness of the body, especially important when one is sick, immobilized or deformed.
• Respect for the individual's needs, giving him or her control over his or her body as a private domain.

Touch in the form of massage can be a

valuable tool in developing children's body image. During infancy, it provides important tactile stimulation. It helps give toddlers body awareness, especially important since boundaries are indefinite. Touch can provide preschoolers with a well-defined body image, which helps with increased motor skills. School age children can use touch to learn positive acceptance of their bodies and boundaries as they begin to relate to others. For example, a seven-year-old girl with a thyroid gland problem was the size of a three-year-old. She was very upset to see how small her size was when someone drew around her body on butcher paper. After receiving massage, however, she remarked that she felt much taller.[1] Adolescents can benefit from touch to reassure them of the integrity of the body, as their body image is in constant change at this age.

Notes

Chapter One
1. Jeanne Hazelton, personal communication with author, January 10, 1992.
2. Julie Fronzuto, intensive care nurse. (Personal communication with author.)
3. Dr. Tiffany Field, "Tactile and Kinesthetic Stimulation Effects on Preterm Neonates," *Pediatrics*, Volume 77, (5) 1986, pp. 654-8.
4. Jake Panskepp, "Of Human Bonding: Social Attachment, Alienation," *Brain-Mind Bulletin*, Volume 5, Number 12, May 5, 1980, p. 2.
5. A. McKechnie et al., "Anxiety States: A Preliminary Report on the Value of Connective Tissue Massage," *Journal of Psychosomatic Research*, Volume 27, Number 2, 1983, pp. 125-9.
6. S. Larson, "Massage With Child and Adolescent Psychiatric Patients" in N. Gunzenhauser, *Advances in Touch*. Skillman, NJ, Pediatric Round Table 14, 1990, pp. 125-32.
7. Robert Coles, "Touching and Being Touched," *The Dial* (Public Broadcasting System publication) December 1980, p. 29.
8. Sidney Jourard, *The Transparent Self*. New York: Van Nostrand Reinhold, 1971, pp. 119-20.
9. James Lynch, *The Broken Heart: The Medical Consequences of Loneliness*. New York: Basic Books, 1977, pp. 135-51.
10. Beth Brothy with Maureen Walsh, "Children Under Stress," *U.S. News & World Report*, October 27, 1986, p. 64.
11. Ibid.
12. Richard Louv, *Childhoods Future: New Hope for the American Family*. Boston: Houghton Mifflin, 1990, p. 15.
13. L. Williams, "Parents and Doctors Fear Growing Misuse of Drug Used to Treat Hyperactive Kids," *Wall Street Journal*, January 15, 1988.
14. Beth Brothy with Maureen Walsh, "Children Under Stress," *U.S. News & World Report*, October 27, 1986, p. 58.
15. Peter Hansen, *The Joy of Stress*. Kansas City: Andrews, McMeel and Parker, 1986, pp. 22-35.
16. C. Schaeffer, H. Hillman, G. Levine, *Therapies for Psychosomatic Disorders in Children*. San Francisco: Jossey-Bass, 1979, pp. xiii-xx.
17. K.J. Roghman, "Daily Stress, Illness, and Use of Health Services in Young Families," *Pediatric Research*, Volume 7, 1973, pp. 520-6.
18. J. Heisel et al., "The significance of life events as contributing factors in the diseases of children," *Journal of Pediatrics*, Volume 83, Number 1, 1973, pp. 119-23.
19. Thomas Verny, *The Secret Life of the Unborn Child*. New York: Summit Books, 1981, p. 210.
20. Lynch, op. cit.

Chapter Two
1. George Downing, *The Massage Book*. New York: Bookworks/Random House, 1972, p. 1.
2. Mary Howell, *Healing at Home*. Boston: Beacon Press, 1978, p. 77.

Chapter Three
1. *Tender Loving Care, Newsletter of International Association of Infant Massage Instructors*, Volume 3, Number 4 (Fall 1987), p. 2.

Chapter Four
1. Mother, quoted in *Tender Loving Care, Newsletter of the International Association of Infant Massage Instructors*, Volume 3, Number 4, Fall 1986.
2. Meir Schneider, *Self Healing: My Life and Vision*. New York: Penguin, 1989.
3. Personal communication with the author.

4. Personal communication with author.
5. Agatha and Calvin Thrash, *Home Remedies*. Scale, AL: Thrash Publications, 1981, p. 124.
6. Robert Pantell, James Fries and Donald Vickery, *Taking Care of Your Child*. Reading, MA: Addison-Wesley, 1977, p. 304.
7. Ibid, p. 356.
8. "The Recuperative Effects of Sports Massage as Compared to Passive Rest," *Massage Therapy Journal*, Vol. 29, No. 1, Winter 1990, pp. 57-66.

Chapter Six
1. Julie Wind, "Massage Therapist Soothes Disabled," *Corvallis Gazette-Times*, July 9, 1991.
2. Kathleen Weber, personal communication, April 1992.
3. Jill Lee, personal communication, April 1992.
4. Dianne Percoraro, "Applications of Massage for Chronic Health Conditions," *Massage Therapy Journal*, Spring 1986, p. 52.
5. Erskine-Milliss and Schonell, "Relaxation Therapy in Asthma: A Critical Review," *Psychosomatic Medicine*, August 1981, pp. 365-70.
6. G. Schwobel, "Psychosomatische therapies des asthma bronchiale," *Anzeim Forsch*, 24 (1948), pp. 481-8.
7. Dr. Cesario Hossri, "The Treatment of Asthma in Children Through Acupuncture Massage," *Journal of American Society of Psychosomatic Dentistry and Medicine*, Volume 23, Number 1, 1976.
8. Nik Waal, "A Special Technique of Psychotherapy in an Autistic Child," *Emotional Problems of Early Childhood*, Caplan, G., editor. New York: Basic Books, 1955, pp. 431-49.
9. Larry Burns-Vidlak, personal communication, April 1989.
10. Jeanne St. John, *High Tech Touch*, p. 57.
11. Martha Welch, *Holding Time*. New York: Simon & Schuster, 1988.
12. R. Smolan, *The Power to Heal*. Englewood Cliffs, NJ: Prentice-Hall, 1990, p. 95.
13. Helen Keller, *The World I Live In*. New York: Methuen Publishing, 1938, p. 39.
14. Meir Schneider, personal communication, May 1989.
15. A 1988 pilot program under Title VI-C (New York State Education Department) found that seventeen children who were both blind and deaf showed a 69 percent increase in language skills after three months of massage. Six blind and deaf children were also evaluated, before and after three months of massage, and found to have a 19 percent increase in sleep time within a 24-hour period. (Evelyn Guyer personal communication, January 20, 1990.)
16. Barbara Von Meyer, personal communication, April 1992.
17. Mother of a seven-year-old boy with mild cerebral palsy, quoted in *High Tech Touch* (Jeanne St. John, editor). Novato, CA: Academic Therapy Publications, 1987, p. 61.
18. Available from the United Cerebral Palsy Center, 2727 Columbine, Denver, CO 80205, (303) 355-7337, $3.00 per copy.
19. Evelyn Guyer, personal communication, January 20, 1990.
20. *Teaching Asanas, An Ananda Marga Manual for Teachers*. Los Altos Hills, CA: Amrit Publications, 1973, p. 233.
21. Kathy Knowles, personal communication, June 1989.
22. Ibid.
23. Kathleen Weber, "Massage for Drug Exposed Infants," *Massage Therapy Journal*, Volume 30, Number 3, 1991, pp. 62-4.
24. Ze'ev Orzech, personal communication, July 10, 1991.
25. D. Safer, "Survey of Medication Treatment for Hyperactive/Inattentive Students," *Journal of the American Medical Association*, Volume 260, Number 15, October 21, 1988, p. 26. D. Connoly et al., "Electromyography Biofeedback on Hyperkinetic Children," *Journal of Biofeedback*, Volume 12, Number 2, 1974, pp. 24-30.
27. Jeanne St. John, *High Tech Touch: Acupressure in the Schools*. Adult level book. Novato, CA: Academic Therapy Publications, 1987, pp. 56-58.
28. Richard Gordon, *Your Healing Hands*. Berkeley, CA: Wingbow Press, 1984, p. 13.
29. L. Arnold, "Hyperactivity With Tactile Defensiveness as a Phobia," *The Journal of School Health*, November 1988, p. 532.
30. S. Henderson et al., "A Hypothesis on the Etiology of Hyperactivity With a Pilot Study Report of Related Drug Therapy," *Pediatrics*, Volume 52, Number 2, 1973.
31. T.C. Hunter, "Massage Therapy—Who Kneads It?", *Arthritis Today*, March-April 1991.
32. Ibid.
33. Diedrich Dasenbrock, personal communication, January 1992.
34. Taylor, R.V., Rimmer, S., Day, B., et al.: "Ascorbic acid supplementation in the treatment of pressure sores," *Lancet* 2:544-546, 1974.
35. *Tender Loving Care*, Volume 4, Number 1, Winter 1988, p. 2.
36. Letter to author, December 17, 1988.
37. Letter to author, January 1989.

Appendix A
1. Reprinted from "The significance of life events as contributing factors in the diseases of children," *Journal of Pediatrics*, Volume 83, Number 1, July 1973, p. 120.

Appendix B
1. Maureen Murdock, *Spinning Inward: Using Guided Imagery With Children for Learning, Creativity & Relaxation*. Boston: Shambhala Publications, 1987, p. 22.
2. Ibid., pp. 20-1.
3. Adapted from *Stress in Childhood*, James H. Humphrey, ed. New York: AMS Press, Inc., 1984, pp. 287-9.

Appendix C
1. Maureen Murdock, *Spinning Inward*. Boston: Shambhala Publications, 1987, pp. 17-19.
2. S. Hunter et al., "Type-A Coronary-Prone Behavior Pattern and Cardiovascular Risk Factor Variables in Children and Adolescents: The Bogalusa Heart Study," *Journal of Chronic Diseases*, Volume 35, 1982, pp. 613-21.
3. Robert Kowalski, *Cholesterol and Children*. New York: Harper & Row, 1988, p. 99.
4. Ibid., p. 8.

Appendix D
1. "Massaging the Handicapped Child," *Tender Loving Care*, Volume 4, Number 1, Winter 1988, p. 2.

Bibliography

Books

Downing, George, *The Massage Book*. New York: Bookworks/ Random House, 1972.

Gordon, Richard, *Your Healing Hands*. Berkeley, CA: Wingbow Press, 1984.

Hansen, Peter, *The Joy of Stress*. Kansas City: Andrews, McMeel and Parker, 1986.

Howell, Mary, *Healing at Home*. Boston: Beacon Press, 1978.

Humphrey, James H., editor, *Stress in Childhood*. New York: AMS Press, Inc., 1984.

Jourard, Sidney, *The Transparent Self*. New York: Van Nostrand Reinhold, 1971.

Keller, Helen, *The World I Live In*. New York: Methuen Publishing, 1938.

Kowalski, Robert, *Cholesterol and Children*. New York: Harper & Row, 1988.

Louv, Richard, *Childhoods Future: New Hope for the American Family*. Boston: Houghton Mifflin, 1990.

Lynch, James, *The Broken Heart: The Medical Consequences of Loneliness*. New York: Basic Books, 1977.

Murdock, Maureen, *Spinning Inward: Using Guided Imagery With Children for Learning, Creativity & Relaxation*. Boston: Shambhala Publications, 1987.

Pantell, Robert, James Fries and Donald Vickery, *Taking Care of Your Child*. Reading, MA: Addison-Wesley, 1977.

St. John, Jeanne, *High Tech Touch: Acupressure in the Schools*. Novato, CA: Academic Therapy Publications, 1987.

Schaeffer, C., H. Hillman, G. Levine, *Therapies for Psychosomatic Disorders in Children*. San Francisco: Jossey-Bass, 1979.

Schneider, Meir, *Self Healing: My Life and Vision*. New York: Penguin, 1989.

Smolan, R., *The Power to Heal*. Englewood Cliffs, NJ: Prentice-Hall, 1990.

Teaching Asanas, An Ananda Marga Manual for Teachers. Los Altos Hills, CA: Amrit Publications, 1973.

Thrash, Agatha and Calvin, *Home Remedies*. Seale, AL: Thrash Publications, 1981.

Verney, Thomas, *The Secret Life of the Unborn Child*. New York: Summit Books, 1981.

Waal, Nik, "A Special Technique of Psychotherapy in an Autistic Child," *Emotional Problems of Early Childhood*, G. Caplan, editor. New York: Basic Books, 1955.

Welch, Martha, *Holding Time*. New York: Simon & Schuster, 1988.

Articles

Arnold, L., "Hyperactivity With Tactile Defensiveness as a Phobia," *The Journal of School Health*, November 1980, p. 532.

Brothy, Beth with Maureen Walsh, "Children Under Stress," *U.S. News & World Report*, October 27, 1986.

Coles, Robert, "Touching and Being Touched," *The Dial* (Public Broadcasting System publication), December 1980.

Connoly, D. et al., "Electromyography Biofeedback on Hyperkinetic Children," *Journal of Biofeedback*, Volume 12, Number 2, 1974.

Erskine-Milliss and Schonell, "Relaxation Therapy in Asthma: A Critical Review," *Psychosomatic Medicine*, August 1981.

Field, Dr. Tiffany, "Tactile and Kinesthetic Stimulation Effects on Preterm Neonates," *Pediatrics*, Volume 77, (5) 1986.

Heisel, J. et al., "The significance of life events as contributing factors in the diseases of children," *Journal of Pediatrics*, Volume 83, Number 1, 1973.

Henderson, A. et al., "A Hypothesis on the Etiology of Hyperactivity With a Pilot Study Report of Related Nondrug Therapy," *Pediatrics*, Volume 52, Number 4, 1973.

Hossri, Dr. Cesario, "The Treatment of Asthma in Children Through Acupuncture Massage," *Journal of American Society of Psychosomatic Dentistry and Medicine*, Volume 23, Number 1, 1976.

Hunter, S. et al., "Type-A Coronary-Prone Behavior Pattern and Cardiovascular Risk Factor Variables in Children and Adolescents: The Bogalusa Heart Study," *Journal of Chronic Diseases*, Volume 35, 1982.

Hunter, T.C., "Massage Therapy—Who Kneads It?", *Arthritis Today*, March-April 1991.

Larson, S., "Massage With Child and Adolescent Psychiatric Patients" in N. Gunzenhauser, *Advances in Touch*. Skillman, NJ, Pediatric Round Table 14, 1990.

"Massaging the Handicapped Child," *Tender Loving Care*, Volume 4, Number 1, Winter 1988.

McKechnie, A. et al., "Anxiety States: A Preliminary Report on the Value of Connective Tissue Massage," *Journal of Psychosomatic Research*, Volume 27, Number 2, 1983.

Panskepp, Jake, "Of Human Bonding: Social Attachment, Alienation," *Brain-Mind Bulletin*, Volume 5, Number 12, May 5, 1980.

Percoraro, Dianne, "Applications of Massage for Chronic Health Conditions," *Massage Therapy Journal*, Spring 1986.

"The Recuperative Effects of Sports Massage as Compared to Passive Rest," *Massage Therapy Journal*, Vol. 29, No. 1, Winter 1990.

Roghman, K.J., "Daily Stress, Illness, and Use of Health Services in Young Families," *Pediatric Research*, Volume 7, 1973.

Safer, D., "Survey of Medication Treatment for Hyperactive/Inattentive Students," *Journal of the American Medical Association*, Volume 260, Number 15, October 21, 1988.

Schwobel, G., "Psychosomatische therapies des asthma bronchiale," *Anzeim Forsch*, 24 (1948).

Taylor, R.V., S. Rimmer, B. Day et al.: "Ascorbic acid supplementation in the treatment of pressure sores," *Lancet* 2:544-546, 1974.

Tender Loving Care, Newsletter of International Association of Infant Massage Instructors, Volume 3, Number 4, Fall 1987, and Volume 4, Number 1, Winter 1988.

Weber, K., "Massage for Drug Exposed Infants," *Massage Therapy Journal*, Volume 30, Number 1, 1991.

Williams, L., "Parents and Doctors Fear Growing Misuse of Drug Used to Treat Hyperactive Kids," *Wall Street Journal*, January 15, 1988.

Wind, Julie, "Massage Therapist Soothes Disabled," *Corvallis Gazette-Times*, July 9, 1991.

Resources

Self-help books

Brenner, Avis. *Helping Children Cope With Stress.* Lexington, MA: D.C. Heath & Co., 1984.

The number and intensity of childhood stresses have dramatically increased in the last decade. This book provides parents, teachers, social workers, nurses, and others with much of the information they need to help children deal with these stresses. Ms. Brenner, an education professor, describes the spectrum of stresses children face and the coping strategies they develop. She distinguishes healthy coping strategies from self-destructive ones. Children need to develop four basic skills for dealing with stress: emotionally close relationships with supportive, caring peers or adults; problem-solving skills; assertiveness; and learning to identify and face stress.

Cohen, Kenneth. *Imagine That! A Child's Guide to Yoga.* Santa Barbara, CA: Santa Barbara Books, 1983.

This book presents yoga postures, relaxation exercises, and meditation for children, to help them develop concentration and release tension and stress from the body. Instructions are written so children can easily understand them, and are accompanied by lovely, colorful illustrations.

Downing, George. *The Massage Book.* New York: Random House, 1972.

This book is an instructional manual of Swedish/Esalen massage for adults. The author gives clear and detailed instructions, and discusses how body tension is related to emotions.

Fassler, J. *Helping Children Cope—Mastering Stress Through Books and Stories.* New York: Free Press, 1978.

This book shows how books and stories can help children cope with specific kinds of stress by reducing their fears and anxieties and encouraging open expression of feelings. It also reviews contemporary children's books about specific stresses, including death, illness, hospitalization, separation fears, divorce, moving, birth of a sibling, and poverty. For each stress, the author lists a child's potential reaction to it, relevant children's books, and questions to help initiate discussion. The emphasis is on books for children in the four- to eight-year age range, but also covers books for older children.

Flaws, Bob. *Turtle Tail and Other Tender Mercies: Traditional Chinese Pediatrics.* Boulder, CO: Blue Poppy Press, 1985.

Chinese medical massage for children (Tuina)

has been practiced from the sixth century A.D. to the present. All traditional Chinese medical hospitals have Tuina departments with rooms set aside for children. This book, by an American practitioner of Chinese medicine, is the first English language text on traditional Chinese pediatrics. It discusses pediatric medical philosophy and history, and the use of diet, Chinese herbs, acupuncture, and Tuina. The author details the basic Tuina manipulations or strokes and specific Tuina treatments for many common children's illnesses, including fever, teething, asthma, earache, colds, whooping cough, tonsilitis, and eczema. *Turtle Tail* is written for American practitioners of Chinese medicine and for parents.

Kuczen, B. *Childhood Stress: Don't Let Your Child Be A Victim.* New York: Delacorte, 1982.

This book, written for parents, provides background information on stress and parental coping; it makes concrete suggestions about minimizing and preventing stress, and controlling and managing it when it occurs.

LeBoyer, Frederick. *Loving Hands.* New York: Alfred A. Knopf, 1981.

Infant massage has been practiced in India for more than two thousand years. Obstetrician and natural birth advocate LeBoyer presents this traditional Indian technique, with directions and lovely photographs.

Miller, S. *Childstress! Understanding and Answering Stress Signals of Infants, Children and Teenagers.* New York: Doubleday & Co., 1982.

The author has seventeen years of experience as a teacher and principal. She discusses stress and stressors in our children today, from birth through teens; the different ways children respond to stress; and concrete suggestions for ways parents and teachers can help children handle stress and avoid creating it. Hundreds of examples from real life situations.

Murdock, Maureen. *Spinning Inward: Using Guided Imagery with Children for Learning, Creativity and Relaxation.* Boston: Shambhala Publications, 1987.

Educator, therapist, and artist Maureen Murdock presents simple exercises in guided imagery for children ages three to eighteen. The exercises are intended to help children relax, focus attention, and increase concentration and creativity. Each chapter presents exercises for a specific goal, such as relaxation, learning with all the senses, positive self image, or improving self-expression.

Pappas, Michael. *Sweet Dreams for Little Ones: Bedtime Fantasies to Build Self-Esteem.* Minneapolis, Minnesota: Winston Press, 1982.

This collection of stories, written by a family counselor, is designed to help children grow closer to their parents and experience both greater relaxation and concentration while being entertained. Each story is preceded by deep breathing and a short massage. The stories themselves stimulate imagination and positive creative fantasy, with the child as the central character.

Prudden, Bonnie. *Pain Erasure the Bonnie Prudden Way.* New York: Ballantine Books, 1982.

Fitness consultant Bonnie Prudden writes on the use of myotherapy, a pressure point massage technique employed to erase trigger points. Prudden claims 95 percent of all pain is related in some way to muscle, and myotherapy helps most pain, including joint pain, facial pain, headaches, menstrual cramps, poor balance, scoliosis, spasticity after brain injury, and sports injuries.

Scholl, Lisette. *Visionetics: The Wholistic Way to Better Eyesight.* New York: Doubleday & Co., 1978.

The author, a yoga and vision improvement teacher, presents a system of vision exercises for all types of vision problems. The exercises are designed to strengthen eye muscles and relax the mind. Eyesight is explained as a reflection of the health of the body, and of the individual's emotional and mental states.

Schneider, M. and Robin, A. *Turtle Manual.* Stony Brook, NY: Psychology Dept., State University of New York, 1979.

This manual for special education teachers combines relaxation training and problem-solving techniques to teach young children with behavior problems to control their own disruptive behavior.

Schneider, Vimala. *Infant Massage: A Handbook for Loving Parents.* New York: Bantam Books, 1982.

The author, a yoga and meditation teacher, shows how to massage a baby using a combination of traditional Indian baby massage and modern Swedish massage. She also discusses the role of massage in promoting infant stimulation, parent-infant bonding, and relaxation training.

Speirer, J., Garty, M., Miller, K., and Martinez, B. *Infant Massage for Developmentally Delayed Babies.* Denver, CO: United Cerebral Palsy Center of Denver, 1984.

This manual teaches Vimala Schneider's infant massage technique with handicapped babies. It discusses the need for touch, along with observations of the benefits of massage to handicapped babies.

St. John, Jeanne. *High Tech Touch: Acupressure in the Schools.* Novato, CA: Academic Therapy Publications, 1987.

This book reports on the use of acupressure massage in a study of twenty-five randomly selected handicapped children; it also gives information on teaching acupressure massage techniques and other exercises to students from primary grades through high school. The author includes sample lesson plans, progress reports, and a detailed bibliography. Schools in several states are currently using these techniques with special education children.

Thrash, Agatha and Calvin. *Home Remedies: Hydrotherapy, Massage, Charcoal, and Other Simple Treatments.* Thrash Publications, Rte. 1, Box 273, Seale, Alabama 36875, 1981.

The authors, one an internist and the other a pathologist, present remedies for many common illnesses and chronic health problems. All the remedies are drugless, and can be used by lay people in the home with very simple equipment. The authors provide detailed scientific rationale for the methods they use.

Welch, Martha. *Holding Time.* New York: Simon and Schuster, 1988.

The author describes her technique, originally used with autistic children, of holding a child to increase attachment between mother and child. She has found that increasing this attachment makes children happier, more co-operative, more self-confident, and less demanding, and increases parental self-confidence and satisfaction.

In-Depth Reading

Touch

Biggar, M. "Maternal Aversion to Mother-Infant Contact," *The Many Facets of Touch*, Catherine Brown, ed. Skillman, NJ: Johnson and Johnson, 1984.

Researchers made detailed observations of 94 mothers with their infants. When mothers consistently disliked physical contact with their three-month-old infants, the children were found to be unusually angry and aggressive at a year old. For example, these infants frequently struck or angrily threatened to strike their mothers in relatively stress-free situations.

Coles, Robert. "Touching and Being Touched," *The Dial* (Public Broadcasting Corporation Publications), December 1980.

Touch is vitally important in communicating with others, offering human connectedness and psychological stability. The author, a child psychiatrist, discusses the experience of American, Eskimo, Brazilian, South African, and Hopi children to substantiate his belief in the positive aspects of touch.

Colton, H. *The Gift of Touch: How Physical Contact Improves Communication, Pleasure and Health.* New York: Putnam, 1983.

Family counselor Colton discusses the deep biological hunger for tactile contact and the need for touch in our lives. Increased touch will lead to better communication among families, friends, colleagues, and strangers, in school, business, and politics, as well as improved physical and psychological well-being. This book contains a good bibliography.

Field, Tiffany et al. "Tactile and Kinesthetic Stimulation Effects on Preterm Neonates," *Pediatrics*, Vol. 77, Number 5, 1986.

This study took place at the University of Miami Medical Center. Twenty premature infants received fifteen-minute massage sessions, three times a day; control premature infants did not. The massaged infants averaged 47 percent greater weight gain per day, were more active and alert, and showed more mature orientation and motor behavior than control infants, and were discharged on the average six days earlier than control infants.

Jourard, Sidney. "An Exploratory Study of Body Accessibility," *British Journal of Social and Clinical Psychology*, Vol. 5, 1966.

The author watched pairs of people talking in coffeeshops in San Juan (Puerto Rico), Paris, London, and Gainesville, Florida, and counted the number of times one person touched another during one hour. The scores were: San Juan, 180; Paris, 110; Gainesville, two; London, none. He also reports on the extent to which college students permit their parents and closest friends of either sex to touch their bodies. His research indicates that hands, arms, shoulders, and the top of the head receive the most contact. Females exchanged more touch with their parents than did males. Most areas of a young adult's body remain untouched unless he or she has a close friend of the opposite sex.

Kulka, A., Fry, C., and Goldstein, F. "Kinesthetic Needs in Infancy," *American Journal of Orthopsychiatry*, Vol. 39, 1960, pp. 562-71.

Three child psychologists report their observations that acute early kinesthetic deprivation causes increased muscle tension in infants, which may lead to hyperactivity or depression in later childhood.

McAnarney, Elizabeth. "Touching and Adolescent Sexuality," *The Many Facets of Touch*, Catherine Brown, ed. Skillman, NJ: Johnson and Johnson, 1984.

This paper explores the link between adolescent pregnancy and touch starvation. Early adolescents (10-14 years of age) are touched less by their parents and their peers than during infancy and childhood. They may engage in sexual intercourse to find the closeness and physical contact they crave, rather than sexual pleasure.

Montagu, Ashley. *Touching: The Human Significance of the Skin*. New York: Harper and Row, 1978.

Montagu, an anthropologist, examines the importance of touching on all aspects of human development. He concludes that touch is a vital necessity throughout life, particularly during infancy and childhood. This book cites hundreds of scientific studies and information culled from scientific works, anecdotes, and quotations from experts in many fields.

Older, J. "A Restoring Touch for Abusing Families," *Child Abuse and Neglect*, Vol. 5, 1981, pp. 487-9.
This article presents a touch exercise used in a support group for abusing and potentially abusing parents. The exercise allows parents to give and receive touch in a relaxing and nonthreatening way. The author reports that although no research has scientifically tested its effects, parents' response has been overwhelmingly positive. At least one mother reported that when she went to hit her baby in a fit of anger, she massaged him instead.

Prescott, J. "Body Pleasure and the Origins of Violence," *The Futurist*, April 1975, pp. 64-74.

Neuropsychologist Prescott examined anthropological data from forty-nine primitive societies. He found that in 73 percent of them, large amounts of physical affection during infancy were correlated with low levels of adult violence, while an absence of such affection corresponded to high levels of violence in adults. He concludes that in order to prevent violence, we need to emphasize touching, holding, and body contact.

Rice, Ruth. "Neurophysiological Development in Premature Infants Following Stimulation," *Journal of Developmental Psychology*, Volume 13, Number 1, 1977.

An experimental group of premature babies received stroking and massage for fifteen minutes, four times daily, over a period of thirty days. The children made significant gains in neurological development, motor development, and weight gain, compared to a control group.

Rosenthal, Maurice. "Psychosomatic Study of Infantile Eczema", *Pediatrics*, Volume 10, 1952, pp. 581-93.

This paper studies the amount of caressing and cuddling given to infants with eczema. Maurice Rosenthal, a pediatrician, hypothesized that in certain predisposed infants, eczema arises because they fail to receive adequate soothing physical contact. He interviewed 25 mothers of infants with eczema and 18 control cases (mothers of infants without eczema), asking both groups whether they picked up their infants when they cried or let the babies "cry it out." Those who commonly let their babies cry were considered to give the children inadequate physical contact. When the mother habitually did nothing for the infant even when it cried, she was considered likely to be reluctant or unable to hold it at other times. By these standards, two thirds of the eczematous infants were found to have inadequate contact, compared to less than one third of the control infants. A sudden decrease in physical contact (caused by abrupt cessation of breastfeeding, mother's health problem, or loss of someone to help with the children) was followed by eczema rather quickly in a number of cases.

Schaffer, H.R., and Emerson, P. "Conflict Over Tactile Experiences in Emotionally Disturbed Children," *Journal of the American Academy of Child Psychology*, Volume 1, 1972, pp. 564-90.

The authors are child psychologists working with severely disturbed children. They believe that when there is a disturbance in tactile stimulation during infancy, children deny their need for it, and begin to fear it instead. They then avoid physical contact by keeping physical distance from others or by creating an elaborate fantasy life.

Shevrin, H. and Toussieng, P. "Patterns of Response to Physical Contact in Early Human Development," *Journal of Child Psychology and Psychiatry*, Volume 5, 1964, pp. 1-13.

Some babies are "cuddlers," desiring close physical contact. "Non-cuddlers" enjoy skin contact and handling, but object to the restriction of movement connected with being held closely. The authors base this conclusion on interviews with the mothers of thirty-seven babies. They believe that the differences between the cuddlers and non-cuddlers are not related to how they are treated by their mothers; all babies enjoy physical contact, but just how they like it is congenitally determined.

Triplett, J. and Arneson, S. "The Use of Verbal and Tactile Comfort to Alleviate Distress in Young Hospitalized Children," *Research in Nursing and Health*, 2 (1979).

Sixty-three children between 3 days and 44 months old—all patients in the pediatric ward of a large Midwestern hospital—were divided into two groups on a random basis. When children in Group A were distressed they were given verbal comfort (talking and singing) for five minutes or until they quieted. Children in Group B were given verbal comfort *and* tactile comfort (patting, stroking, rocking, and holding). In 40 verbal-only interventions (Group A) only 7 succeeded in quieting the children, but in 60 verbal-tactile interventions (Group B), 53 were successful. This indicates that tactile comfort is the distressed child's method of choice.

Massage
Downes, A., editor. "Massaging the Handicapped Child," *Tender Loving Care: the Newsletter of the International Association of Infant Massage Instructors*, Volume 4, Number 1, 1985.

This special issue features three articles on massaging the handicapped child, including children with tactile defensiveness, prematurity, cerebral palsy, and spina bifida. Some specific children and their treatments are discussed.

Klaus, Marshall H. and Phyllis H. Klaus. *The Amazing Newborn*. Menlo Park, CA: Addison-Wesley, 1985.

This book illustrates the special capacities with which babies begin life. Of special interest is the mention of a study by French pediatricians Amiel-Tison and Grenier. Both arms and the neck work together to keep babies' heads from falling, so that unless the neck muscles are very relaxed, very young babies cannot reach out. Amiel-Tison and Grenier found that one out of two newborns could reach for objects after their necks were rubbed for three to five minutes, which caused the neck muscles to relax.

Martin, G. "Trauma and Recall in Massage: A Personal Experience," *The Massage Journal*, Winter 1985.

Martin, a massage therapist, writes of massage triggering her recall of a terribly traumatic childhood injury. The trauma and fear associated with her injury had been stored in her chest and were released during the chest massage. Ms. Martin gives examples of massage stimulating recall in other individuals.

McKechnie, A., et al. "Anxiety States: A Preliminary Report on the Value of Connective Tissue Massage," *Journal of Psycho-somatic Research*, Vol. 27, no. 2, 1983.

This pilot study used massage to treat patients with a history of severe anxiety and difficulty relaxing. After ten sessions of back massage, objective tests showed a decrease in levels of anxiety and bodily tensions.

Mitchell, R. "Is Kneading Needed?" *Developmental Medical Child Neurology*, Volume 18, Number 1 (1976).

In an editorial, the author reports on baby massage in Russia, where mothers massage their babies daily and baby massage is an accepted and universally practiced part of child care. Mothers and doctors believe it makes the body and limbs supple, strengthens and tones the muscles and skin, and generally increases the infant's well-being. The babies thoroughly enjoy it. The author concludes by urging a controlled study to establish whether massaged babies have any advantage over unmassaged babies.

Schutz, Will and Evelyn Turner. *Body Fantasy*. New York: Harper and Row, 1976.

Rolfing is a specialized method of deep massage. Psychotherapist Schutz combined rolfing and guided fantasy in the therapy of Turner, a middle-aged woman. Their account of the treatment demonstrates how childhood experiences became incorporated in the body; as chronic physical tension was released, childhood memories and repressed emotional conflicts came to the surface.

Teeguarden, Ilona. "Acupressure in the Classroom," *East West Journal*, August 1985.

Jin Shin Do acupressure is a form of pressure point massage using the principles of acupuncture that focuses on deep release of tension. It is also a form of therapeutic touch, giving the individual the feeling of being held, cradled, and safe. This article reports on the effects of Jin Shin Do when it was used by the Santa Cruz County (California) Office of Education. Twenty-five randomly selected handicapped children received eight weekly hour-long Jin Shin Do sessions. They showed a decrease of tension and improvement in social and emotional behavior and health. Motor, cognitive, and communication skills increased. The author cites the cases of specific children with problems such as moderate retardation, hyperactivity, and autism.

Waal, Nik. "A Special Technique of Psychotherapy in an Autistic Child," *Emotional Problems in Early Infancy*, Caplan, G., editor. New York: Basic Books, 1955.

The author, a psychiatrist, discusses how she successfully treated an autistic child, using massage to achieve healthy emotional adjustment and release of tension.

Children and Stress
Bedell, J., et al. "Life Stress and the Psychological and Medical Adjustment of Chronically Ill Children," *Journal of Psychosomatic Research*, Volume 21, 1977, pp. 237-42.

The authors investigated the relationship between life stress and the day-to-day psychological and physical well-being of chronically ill children. These children between the ages of 6 and 15 attended a 3-week residential summer camp. They were given objective psychological tests to assess the amount of life stress in the previous 12 months, their self-concept, and their anxiety levels. The study related their health problems to their chronic ailments, and concluded that children with low levels of stress had a better self-concept and significantly fewer health problems related to their chronic disease than high-stress children.

Cheek, D. "Maladjustment Patterns Apparently Related to Imprinting at Birth," *American Journal of Clinical Hypnosis*, Volume 18, Number 2, 1975.

Using information obtained through reviewing birth memories under hypnosis, this article discusses how maternal pain and emotional distress at birth can cause conditioned responses in later life. (For example, one patient had migraine headaches initiated by a high forceps delivery.) These conditioned responses may change as the initial memory is exposed to conscious reasoning and later perspective during age regression hypnosis.

Elkind, David. *Hurried Children: Growing Up Too Fast Too Soon.* Menlo Park, CA: Addison-Wesley, 1981.

The author, a child psychologist, discusses how schools, media, and changing family structures push modern children into achievement and adult responsibilities for which they are not ready. The book discusses the negative effects of hurrying, including psychosomatic illness and lifelong negative patterns of stress reaction.

Heisel, J., et al. "Significance of Life Events as Contributing Factors in the Diseases of Children," *Journal of Pediatrics,* Volume 83, Number 1, 1973.

A study of five groups of children examined the social-psychological events that occurred in their environment before the onset of illness. The five groups: children with rheumatoid arthritis, children hospitalized for hernia or appendix surgery, children with psychiatric problems, general pediatric patients, and hemophiliacs. Twice as many of the sick children experienced major life changes (stresses) as would have been expected in a control population of healthy children.

Humphrey, J., editor. *Stress in Childhood.* New York: AMS Press, 1984.

This is a collection of articles covering causes of childhood stress, how children react emotionally, physically, and behaviorally to stress, and how to control and reduce stress in childhood. For health professionals who work with children.

Hunter, S.M. "Coping Behavior and Blood Pressure in Youth," *Circulation,* Volume 68, Number 4, 1983.

This biracial study of 371 children ages 8-17 found a significant correlation between how they coped with problems and their blood pressure. Children with high blood pressure tended to cope with problems by denying they existed, whereas children with normal blood pressure tended to find and apply solutions to problems.

Hunter, S.M., et al. "Type A Coronary-Prone Behavior Patterns in Children and Adolescents," *Journal of Chronic Disease,* Volume 35, Number 8, 1982.

This biracial study of 400 children ages 8-17 investigated the relationship between Type A and Type B behavior and cholesterol level in the blood. Children filled out a questionnaire, rating themselves on 17 items (such as restlessness, hurriedness, being hard-driving, and expression of feelings). Those who showed high degrees of Type A behavior had significantly higher blood cholesterol levels than Type B children. This finding is important because adults with high cholesterol levels are statistically more likely to have coronary artery disease. The Type A children had louder voice patterns, walked and ate faster, performed more rapidly on a perceptual motor task, and were more competitive than the Type B children.

Researchers also found that boys and girls who believed that there were societal blockages for their achievement (such as their race and sex) had higher blood pressure than those who did not feel this way.

Leitch, M. and Escalona, S. "The Reaction of Infants to Stress" in *The Psychoanalytic Study of the Child,* Volumes 3-4. New York: International University Press, 1949, pp. 121-40.

Two child psychologists discuss their observations of infants. Under stress, infants show changes in posture, motility, activity level, readiness to startle, breathing, circulation, social responsiveness and attention span. Different temperaments react differently to stress. Case histories are included.

Lynch, James J. *The Broken Heart: The Medical Consequences of Loneliness.* New York: Basic Books, 1977.

This book presents statistical and clinical evidence that long-lasting human relationships are important conditions for emotional and physical health. The negative impact of adult loneliness on virtually every major disease is discussed, as well as how loneliness during childhood can contribute to the subsequent development of various physical diseases.

The author also presents his own research on touch and the heart. Two separate studies, one in a cardiac intensive care unit and the other in a shock-trauma unit, monitored patients' electrocardiograms during a simple touch, the taking of the pulse. Both studies showed that touch had dramatic effects on the heart, notably normalizing heart rate and rhythm. It had this effect on patients of all ages, including those in comas or near death.

Powell, G.F., Brasel, J.A. and Blizzard, R.M. "Emotional Deprivation and Growth Retardation Simulating Idiopathic Hypopituitarism," *New England Journal of Medicine*, Vol. 276, No. 23, 1967.

This article by three physicians discusses the treatment of 13 children for growth retardation caused by emotional deprivation. Their home environment was very poor; the authors called it "hostile child rearing." This stress caused lowered pituitary gland functioning and slow growth. When placed in a convalescent hospital, they began to grow rapidly, despite a lack of medication and psychiatric treatment.

Roghman, K.J. "Daily Stress, Illness, and Use of Health Services in Young Families," *Pediatric Research*, Volume 7, 1973.

512 mothers kept a diary for a month; they recorded the occurence in the family of stressful events, illness, and use of health services. The study defined stress as any event that the family perceived as upsetting, excepting illness. Examples included loss of job, marital discord or divorce, police contacts, death in the family, arguments over children's behavior, financial worries, or problems with employers or neighbors. Researchers found that the probability of minor illness such as fevers, coughs, headaches, and colds doubled for mothers and increased 50 percent for children on a stressful day. This study is evidence that increased childhood illness related to stress happens in the event of minor illnesses and short-term stress as well as major illness or long-term stress.

Williams, L. "Parents and Doctors Fear Growing Misuse of Drug Used to Treat Hyperactive Kids," *Wall Street Journal*, Jan. 15, 1988.

This article reports on the controversy over the use of the medication Ritalin to treat hyperactivity. On one side are those who say that Ritalin is a godsend; it enables hypertensive children to concentrate and control their impulses so that they can do schoolwork. On the other side, increasing numbers of parents and professionals fear that the drug substitutes for more productive ways to help children whose discipline problems stem from other causes, including minor brain damage and the stress of growing up too early. Stress may cause children to be aggressive and inattentive. Ritalin was prescribed for 750,000 children in 1989, six times the 1971 figure. It has a number of side effects including insomnia, nervousness, growth suppression, and dizziness. According to child psychologist David Elkind, "Drugs should be the treatment of last resort, but Ritalin is convenient. Let's face it: it solves the problem."

Children and Relaxation Training

Anneberg, L. "A Study of the Different Relaxation Techniques in Tactile Deficient and Tactile Defensive Children" (Masters Thesis, University of Kansas, 1973).

The author begins by discussing how important proper tactile functioning is for children's physical, mental, emotional, and social development. She then summarizes her research into the effect of relaxation training on tactile defensiveness (fear of touch), and on decreased tactile perception, in children ages four through eleven. She concludes that progressive relaxation and/or autogenic training increased tactile perception, and decreased tactile defensiveness.

McBrien, R. "Using Relaxation With First Grade Boys," *Elementary School Guidance and Counseling*, February 1978.

This article is a case history of relaxation training with a hyperactive first-grade boy. Over a three-month period the boy learned progressive relaxation and imagery; he was then able to voluntarily relax his whole body, and use his relaxation skills to achieve self-management of his hyperactivity.

Richter, I., et al. "Cognitive and Relaxation Treatment of Pediatric Migraine," *Pain*, Vol. 25, 1986.

This study compared the effectiveness of two active treatments, relaxation training and cognitive coping, with a placebo control in the treatment of 42 children and adolescents with migraine. Their ages ranged from nine to eighteen years; each had suffered from migraine for at least two years. (Children with allergic, purely dietary, or menstrual headache were excluded, as were those with unstable emotional or medical problems likely to require other medical intervention.)

The children were placed in one of three groups: relaxation training, cognitive coping, or control. All children were tested for anxiety and depression to insure the control group had equivalent amounts. The relaxation training group was taught deep breathing and sequential tensing and relaxing of large muscle groups to achieve total body relaxation. They were told to practice daily and use their relaxation skills during stress or at the onset of a headache. The cognitive coping group was taught to change maladaptive thought processes which produce unpleasant emotions which in turn may precipitate a headache. They learned fantasy, simple problem solving, awareness of the effects of thinking upon emotions, and daily monitoring of stress reactions. The control group was taught only to recognize and label their emotions and to discuss their feelings daily with a parent or friend. After six weeks of training, both active groups reported less severe headaches. Children with the most severe headaches reported their headaches were now less severe. The control group showed no improvement in headache frequency or severity. The two active groups continued to improve through a follow-up sixteen weeks later; the control group did not.

Russell, H. and Carter, J. "Biofeedback Training With Children: Consultation, Questions, Applications and Alternatives," *Journal of Clinical Child Psychology*, Volume 23, Spring 1978.

Children with biofeedback relaxation training can learn to significantly influence their behavior by controlling their own physiological functioning. This article provides examples of such behavior, including mental, emotional, and physical problems. The authors are child psychologists who use biofeedback with children. They discuss their own research, which indicates that as children become more relaxed through biofeedback training, they learn better in the classroom.

Schaeffer, C., Millman, H., and Levine, G. *Therapies for Psychosomatic Disorders in Children*. San Francisco: Jossey-Bass, Inc., 1979.

This book presents treatment modes for many psychosomatic disorders, including behavior modification, psychotherapy, relaxation training and decreasing muscle tension with biofeedback. It is quite technical, and not designed for parents.

Volpe, R. "Feedback Facilitated Relaxation Training in School Counseling," *Canadian Counselor*, Volume 9, Number 3/4, June 1975.

This paper provides a rationale for school counselors to use biofeedback training to help children learn relaxation skills. The author's research indicates that children as young as six years of age can learn relaxation skills with biofeedback. He discusses some of the childhood conditions that have been successfully treated this way, including phobias, stuttering and stammering, test anxiety, tension in autistics, hyperactivity, and poor fine-motor control accompanying cerebral palsy. He believes relaxation training can help children learn better, cope better, and provide an alternative for the use of tranquilizers now being given to as many as 200,000 North American children.

Miscellaneous

Bates, T. and E. Grunwaldt. "Myofascial Pain in Childhood," *Journal of Pediatrics*, Vol. 22, No. 4, 1952.

Two pediatricians report on their eight years of treating childhood skeletal myofascial pain, associated with painful muscle spasm but not connected with abnormal neurological disease or evidence of bone or joint disease. Spasms may result from sudden trauma, chronic repetitive strain, or prolonged chilling, with acute and chronic infections and fatigue among the predisposing factors. Myofascial pain is quite common among children, but often is discovered only by carefully questioning the child. In each muscle group involved there is at least one small hypersensitive "trigger area." The trigger area is located by using firm but gentle fingertip pressure, which will elicit deep burning local pain and referred pain over a larger area; this is the location of the pain for which the child has been brought to the physician. Stimulating the trigger area causes a pattern of referred pain which does not vary significantly from patient to patient.

The trigger area may be treated by ethyl chloride spray or injection of procaine hydrochloride. A very small amount of ethyl chloride spray is applied over the entire trigger area as the muscles in the area of pain reference are gently massaged and stretched. (The authors do not report on the use of massage rather than spray to treat the trigger area, but it can be highly effective. For more on trigger point massage, see *Pain Erasure* by Bonnie Prudden, q.v.)

The authors treated eighty-five cases of skeletal myofascial pain, in ages from 14 months to 17 years. One 3-year-old boy had severe calf pains which caused a serious sleep problem (five episodes of screaming at night and poor napping). He first began to complain of leg pains at 2½. Treatment of trigger areas in knees, thighs and calf areas was done four times at two-day intervals using ethyl chloride spray. The child complained no more of pain and slept well at nap and night time. Other examples of successful treatments were: 1) trigger areas causing pain and limitation of motion in the legs in a 3-year-old girl, three months after having polio, 2) trigger areas causing severe prostrating headaches with nausea, vertigo, and vomiting in a 9-year-old boy. These cases could have been successfully treated with massage rather than spray. Out of the 85 cases, there was complete relief of pain in 71 cases and some relief in 9 cases.

Blaesing, S., and Brockhause, J. "The Development of Body Image in the Child," *Nursing Clinics of North America*, Vol. 7, No. 4, December 1972.

This article by two nursing instructors discusses what constitutes body image (the child's mental self-image), how it develops from infancy through the teen years, and its importance. The child's concept of his body image is a primary indicator of his degree of personality organization and ego strength. If it is not definite and relatively stable, the child cannot perceive self or others accurately, or test reality adequately; the result is severe anxiety and difficulty interacting with the environment. Tactile stimulation is critically important in developing healthy body image; some ways to provide it are rocking, holding, massaging, and water play. Parents' or other caregivers' attitudes toward the body, conveyed verbally or non-verbally, make an indelible impression on the child's concept of his body and its functions. Children who are accepted by their parents usually do not undervalue or overvalue their bodies. The more emotionally disturbed a child is, the less tolerant he is of his physical self. Any body area about which the child is emotionally conflicted will tend to be distorted in the body image; for example, the child may see it as larger, smaller, or differently shaped than it really is. Children who have a negative body image often have a great need for physical stimulation.

Clarke, Ann M. and A.D. Clarke, eds. *Early Experience: Myth and Evidence*. New York: Free Press, 1976.

The authors, educational psychologists, offer case studies and scientific research to support their thesis that a child's personality is far from wholly shaped during the formative years of early childhood. Even severely deprived or stressed children can flourish mentally, emotionally, and socially if they are later given a nourishing and stimulating environment.

Klaus, Marshall H. and J. Kennel. *Parent-Infant Bonding*. St. Louis: Mosby, 1982.

Mothers and their premature infants often have difficulty becoming attached to each other after a separation. Pediatricians Klaus and Kennel studied parent-infant bonding based on this observation. They concluded that when there is early and extended mother-baby contact in the first few days of life, compared to a lack of such contact, mothers are more affectionate, more successful in breastfeeding, more soothing, touch their babies more, and make more eye-to-eye contact. Also, their babies' weight gain is greater, and at age 3½ their IQ is higher.

The authors also survey other investigators' research. Infants who have had long separations from their parents are three to four times more likely to be battered or neglected children than children who were not separated from their parents. In other mammals, if the young are not present during the initial bonding period, maternal behavior quickly disapppears. The last chapters of the book discuss how health care professionals can best care for the parents of premature, sick, deformed, stillborn, or dead infants.

Lynch, James J. *The Language of the Heart: The Body's Response to Human Dialogue.* New York: Basic Books, 1986.

The entire cardiovascular system responds when we communicate with others by talking and listening. The entire body is activated when one speaks, through changes in blood pressure, heart rate and activity, and blood flow to different areas. This book describes the scientific discovery of this response. This research implies that disturbed communication causes disrupted relationships, which lead to emotional isolation and serious medical problems. Improved communication can have dramatic positive effects on personal relationships and health.

Magid, Ken and Carole A. McElvey. *High Risk: Children Without a Conscience.* New York: Bantam Books, 1987.

The central thesis of this book is that there is a strong link between criminality and a lack of proper emotional attachment between children and their parents. This attachment begins in infancy and continues to form during childhood; it is essential for formation of a healthy personality. Breaks in attachment may result from many factors (such as child neglect or abuse, poor daycare arrangements, teen pregnancy, foster care, loss of a parent, and divorce) but are most devastating during infancy.

The long-term consequences of failure to form an affectional bond include an inability to establish and maintain deep interpersonal relationships, deep-seated hostility and rage, and often the creation of a psychopathic personality. Psychopaths make up a significant proportion of psychoses or criminals, and have a huge impact on society. They are literally people without a conscience. The least bonded or attached children become the most extreme psychopaths, exemplified by Charles Manson and Ted Bundy. The authors believe that social problems contribute to a national attachment crisis, and that many more psychopathic personalities will be created unless our nation changes its strategies on adoption, daycare, and child abuse and neglect. Adequate attention must be given to the needs of children and families, and especially to the importance of emotional attachment.

Schneider, Meir, *Self-Healing: My Life and Vision.* London: Routledge and Kegan Paul, 1987.

An account by Dr. Meir Schneider of his life and the development of his therapeutic body work technique, called Self-Healing. He recovered from congenital blindness using the Bates (*Better Eyesight Without Glasses*) method. He then used his discovery of the body's healing power to develop Self-Healing. His technique combines massage, movement, breathing, and mental imagery. Dr. Schneider has worked with thousands of adults and children, many with physical problems ranging from chronic pain, eye problems, and muscular dystrophy to polio and rheumatoid arthritis. Many have shown dramatic improvement. For Dr. Schneider's address, see References.

Samuels, Mike, and Samuels, Nancy. *The Well Child Book: Your Child From Four to Twelve.* New York: Simon and Schuster, 1982.

This manual provides clear, up-to-date, and comprehensive information. There are three sections: preventive medicine for parents; anatomy and physiology for children; common illness and accidents, for parents and children. The first section explains particularly well how stress can affect children's health, and how social support, parenting styles, and relaxation techniques can reduce stress. The authors report that social supports have been found to protect people from illness during stressful times.

Watson, J. *Psychological Care of the Infant and Child.* Boston: W.W. Norton and Company, 1932.

Dr. John Watson was the Dr. Spock of his time, an extremely influential pediatrician in the 1920s and '30s; much of the material in this book was originally published in *McCall's.* His advice on the dangers of coddling, mother love, and physical contact helped create the idea that touching was "spoiling," created dependent personalities, and was to be avoided at all costs. Dr. Watson recognized the power of touch to soothe and comfort children, but advised against it. "Never hug and kiss them, never let them sit in your lap. If you must, kiss them once on the forehead when they say goodnight. Shake hands with them in the morning." Thumbsucking, while soothing, was to be discouraged by fingerless mittens, painting bitter aloe on the fingers, scolding, or rapping the fingers sharply. This book is of interest because it shows how the association between touching and spoiling began, and how parents were first discouraged from touching their children.

Audio-Visual Educational Materials

Expectations—A Story About Stress, from Walt Disney Educational Media Company, 500 S. Buena Vista, Burbank, CA 91521; (800) 423-2555. Film: $529.00; video: $397.00.

This film is designed for classroom use. It helps pre-adolescents recognize the causes and symptoms of stress, and stimulates discussion about methods of dealing with stress.

Family Relaxation and Self Control Program (two volumes, 3 cassettes each), from Future Health, Inc., 975A Briston Pike, Bensalem, PA 19020; (215) 639-2340. $29.95 per volume.

The Feldenkrais Resource Catalogue, PO Box 2067, Berkeley, CA 94702; 1-800-765-1907. Audio tapes, video tapes, and books on the "Awareness Through Movement" or Feldenkrais Method.

Gentle Places and Quiet Spaces Catalog, published twice yearly by the Conscious Living Foundation, PO Box 9, Drain, OR 97435; 1-800-752-2256. Single copies free. For copies of twenty or more, 10 cents each.

This catalog features a variety of relaxation aids for adults and children. Available for children are coloring workbooks on relaxation, and cassette tapes on deep muscle relaxation, lullabies, bedtime stories, and how to deal with stress.

International Association of Infant Massage Instructors, PO Box 16103, Portland, OR 97216.

IAIMI maintains a directory of infant massage instructors in the United States and abroad. Its newsletter, *Tender Loving Care,* is published four times yearly and covers a range of material related to infant massage. Past issues have discussed massage for the handicapped child, massage for prematures and aaopted babies, book reviews and updates from instructors, and comments from parents.

Keeping in Touch, from Morel Media, 114 W. Cresent Ln/PO Box F, Stelle, IL 60919. Cost: $69.95.

Maria and Wayne Mathias are massage instructors. Their sixty-minute video teaches parents how to massage babies, older children, and teenagers. It features relaxation techniques for parents and children and thirty different massage strokes. Comes in VHS and Beta format.

Kiddie QR (Quieting Reflex) and *Quieting Reflex for Adolescents: A Choice,* from Quieting Reflex Publications, 119 Forrest Dr, Wethersfield, CT 06109.

Kiddie QR includes: Introductory booklet; four audio cassettes; four booklets containing 100 pages of transcript of tapes; instruction guide. $59.50.

Quieting Reflex for Adolescents: A Choice includes: 38-page manual; four audio cassettes; teaching suggestions. $69.50.

Kiddie QR and *Quieting Reflex for Adolescents* are educational preventive health care programs. They are designed to train children to deal with stress and get rid of excess tension. Both programs are divided into sixteen brief (three- to seven-minute) experimental exercises, and are designed to be integrated into classroom use, or dental and pediatric settings. The authors are a classroom teacher and a psychiatrist. Applications for healthy children, children with psychosomatic complaints, and special needs children are discussed. QR has been successfully incorporated into health curricula from first grade through high school.

Loving Hands, from New Yorker films, 43 W 61st St, New York, NY 10023. $325.00.

This 16mm film by Frederick LeBoyer is a lyric treatment of Indian baby massage, featuring an Indian mother massaging her baby.

The Touch Film: With Dr. Jessie Porter, from Sterling Productions, 1609 Sherman Av #201, Evanston, IL 60201; (312) 475-4445. $395.00 purchase; $60.00 rental; free preview.

This 22-minute film is a lecture by psychologist Jessie Potter, interspersed with pointed and humorous vignettes. It discusses how American children are touched and taught to touch others, and the different ways male and female children are taught about touch. Potter discusses the repercussions this can have in adult relationships. The film also covers touch deprivation in adulthood and old age, and makes a strong case for affectionate supportive touch throughout life.

Touching, from Psychological Films, 110 N Wheeler St, Orange, CA 92669; (714) 639-4646. Film: $400.00 purchase, $40.00 rental; video: $350.00.
   This film, made from the book *Touching*, discusses the importance of touch throughout life. It is alternately moving, hilarious, and inspiring. Includes interviews with Dr. Ashley Montagu.

Working with Your Special Child: Massage, Movement, and Water for Spastic Quadriplegia (video tape), from Leonore Horden, PO Box 2247, Roseburg, Oregon 97470; (503) 672-7001.

Instructors

Larry Burns-Vidlak is an expert on massage therapy for the disabled. He is available for lectures and workshops on this topic, and will have instructional videos and a book available in the near future. Contact: Larry Burns-Vidlak, 3620 N. 38th St., Phoenix, AZ 85018.

Helen Campbell is a social worker and massage therapist, an expert on massage for the catastrophically and terminally ill. She lectures and leads workshops on this topic, and is currently writing a book as well. Contact: Helen Campbell, 2835 Adeline Dr., Burlingame, CA 94010-5969.

Loretta Englehardt, Ph.D. c/o Leadership, Training, and Evaluation Associates, Inc., PO Box 751, Spearfish, SD 57783 (605-642-4795). Dr. Englehardt is the originator of a program called Awareness and Relaxation Through Biofeedback, which was introduced in the two elementary, junior and senior high schools in Spearfish, South Dakota. Students were taught muscle relaxation skills through biofeedback, to decrease anxiety (improving academic performance) and raise self-

esteem. The program proved to be educationally and statistically significant. Dr. Englehardt, a nurse, psychotherapist, and biofeedback specialist, is available to conduct one- or two-day workshops in awareness, relaxation, and biofeedback techniques. These workshops are for conselors of children from kindergarden through high school, and for educators.
   Workshop cost: $400 per day plus expenses.

The Feldenkrais Guild provides information on Feldenkrais instructors in the United States and abroad. 524 Ellsworth St, PO Box 489, Albany OR 97321 (503-926-0981).

Mary Gengler-Fuhr is a pediatric occupational therapist and infant massage instructor. She teaches workshops for other health care professionals working with special needs children, called *A Neurophysiological Approach to Infant Massage*. Contact: Pediatric Therapy Services, 14104—76th Ave. E., Puyallup, WA 98373.

Dr. Meir Schneider is the author of *Self-Healing: My Life and Vision* (q.v.). He teaches his technique, called Self-Healing, to healthy individuals and those with health problems or physical handicaps. He has pamphlets and audiotapes available. Contact: Center for Self-Healing, 1718 Taraval St., San Francisco, CA 94116.

Dr. Jeanne St. John is the author of *High Tech Touch: Acupressure in the Schools* (q.v.). She is available for lectures and workshops on the therapeutic use of acupressure with children, and how to begin an acupressure program in a public school. Contact: Jeanne St. John, Ph.D., 809 Bay Ave., Capitola, CA 95010.

Robert Toporek specializes in Rolfing children. He is available for lectures or demonstrations on this topic, and has made a video of his work. Contact PO Box 30279, Philadelphia, PA 19103.

Index

Checklists of Strokes for a Full Body Massage

Back (page 16)
✓ Basic relaxation sequence.
✓ Apply oil or lotion.
✓ Back warmer ten times.
✓ Raking the back three times.
✓ Back warmer three times.
✓ Kneading the shoulders one minute.
✓ Back warmer three times.
✓ Thumbstroking the lower back one minute.
✓ Kneading the buttocks one minute.
✓ Back warmer three times.
✓ Thumbstroking between the shoulder blades one minute.
✓ Back warmer ten times.
✓ Basic relaxation sequence.

Back of the Leg (page 19)
✓ Basic relaxation sequence.
✓ Apply oil or lotion.
✓ Leg warmer ten times.
✓ Raking the back of the leg one minute.
✓ Leg warmer three times.
✓ Thumbstroking the sole of the foot one minute.
✓ Circle the ankle bones six times.
✓ Leg warmer three times.
✓ Thumbstroking the back of the leg one minute.
✓ Leg warmer ten times.
✓ Basic relaxation sequence.

Head, Neck and Shoulders (page 22)
✓ Basic relaxation sequence.
✓ Apply oil or lotion.
✓ Head warmer ten times.
✓ Diagonal neck stroke ten times.
✓ Head warmer three times.
✓ Scalp circles one minute.
✓ Head warmer three times.
✓ Forehead and eye circles three times.
✓ Face warmer six times.
✓ Cheek circles thirty seconds
✓ Head warmer ten times.
✓ Basic relaxation sequence.

Chest and Stomach (page 26)
✓ Basic relaxation sequence.
✓ Apply oil or lotion.
✓ Front warmer ten times.
✓ Heart warmer ten times.
✓ Front warmer three times.
✓ Stomach warmer three times.
✓ Stomach smoother thirty seconds.
✓ Kneading the stomach one minute.
✓ Front warmer ten times.
✓ Basic relaxation sequence.

Arm (page 29)
✓ Basic relaxation sequence.
✓ Apply oil or lotion.
✓ Arm warmer ten times.
✓ Thumbstroking the inside of the arm one minute.
✓ Arm warmer three times.
✓ Raking the outside of the arm one minute.
✓ Arm warmer three times.
✓ Hand friction thirty seconds.
✓ Thumbstroking the back of the hand thirty seconds.
✓ Thumbstroking the palm thirty seconds.
✓ Stretching the fingers three times for each finger.
✓ Arm warmer ten times.
✓ Basic relaxation sequence.

Front of the Leg (page 33)
✓ Basic relaxation sequence.
✓ Apply oil or lotion.
✓ Leg warmer ten times.
✓ Raking the front of the leg one minute.
✓ Leg warmer three times.
✓ Foot friction fifteen seconds.
✓ Thumbstroking the top of the foot thirty seconds.
✓ Stretch and stroke the toes three times for each toe.
✓ Leg warmer ten times.
✓ Basic relaxation sequence.

Copy this page and place it where you can easily refer to it when you're working with your child.